15 MINUTE
WORKOUT FOR WOMEN

Everyday Pilates
by Alycea Ungaro

Abs Workout
by Joan Pagano

Better Back Workout
by Suzanne Martin

Total Body Workout
by Joan Pagano

Gentle Yoga
by Louise Grime

London, New York, Melbourne, Munich, and Delhi

Senior Editor Jennifer Latham
Senior Art Editor Susan Downing
Editorial Assistant Erin Boeck Motum
Managing Editor Dawn Henderson
Managing Art Editor Christine Keilty
Art Director Peter Luff
Publisher Mary-Clare Jerram

Stills Photography Ruth Jenkinson
DTP Designer Sonia Charbonnier
Senior Production Controller Alice Holloway
Senior Production Editor Jennifer Murray
Senior Jacket Creative Nicola Powling
US Editor Rebecca Warren

DVD produced for Dorling Kindersley by
Chrome Productions www.chromeproductions.com

This edition produced for The Book People,
Hall Wood Avenue, Haydock, St. Helens WA11 9UL

This edition published in 2013
First published in Great Britain in 2010
by Dorling Kindersley Limited
80 Strand, London WC2R 0RL
Penguin Group (UK)

2 4 6 8 10 9 7 5 3 1
001–192907–Jan/13

Material in this publication was previously published by DK
in *15 Minute Everyday Pilates*, 2008; *15 Minute Abs Workout*,
2009; *15 Minute Better Back Workout*, 2008; *15 Minute Total
Body Workout*, 2008; and *15 Minute Gentle Yoga*, 2008.

Health warning
All participants in fitness activities must assume the
responsibility for their own actions and safety. If you have
any health problems or medical conditions, consult with
your physician before undertaking any of the activities set
out in this book. The information contained in this book
cannot replace sound judgement and good decision
making, which can help reduce risk of injury.

A CIP catalogue record for this
book is available from the
British Library

ISBN 978-1-4093-2790-5

Printed and bound in China by
Leo Paper Products Ltd.

Discover more at
www.dk.com

MD Coaches Frances — 028 3833 9397

contents

>> **safety** issues

Before you start any training programme, you must make sure that it is safe for you to begin. First, take the PAR-Q questionnaire on the opposite page to see if you should check with your doctor before beginning. Remember, it's always wise to consult your doctor if you're suffering from an illness or any injuries.

Test your fitness

When starting a fitness programme, it's useful to see how your muscular fitness measures up by counting how many repetitions you can perform or how many seconds you can hold a contraction. The three exercises shown here will assess your muscular endurance in the lower, middle, and upper body. Record your results, noting the date, and after three months of training, repeat the tests. When you reassess yourself, perform the same version of the exercise. Before attempting the exercises, warm up first by moving briskly for five minutes.

If you are just beginning to exercise, or coming back to it after a long break, you may prefer to perform your first assessment after two or three months of exercising on a regular basis.

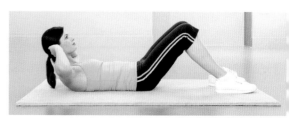

Middle body   *Crunch with Scoop*
Count how many crunches you can do consecutively without resting. This is not a full sit-up. Lift your head and shoulders no higher than 30 degrees off the mat.

Your score

Excellent	50 reps or more
Good	35–49 reps
Fair	20–34 reps
Poor	20 reps or less

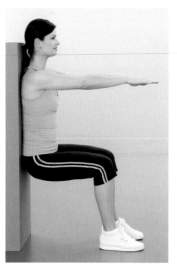

Lower body

Wall Squat
Slide down until your thighs are parallel to the floor and hold the position for as long as you can. (If you cannot slide all the way down, go as far as you can.)

Your score

Excellent	90 seconds or more
Good	60 seconds
Fair	30 seconds
Poor	less than 30 seconds

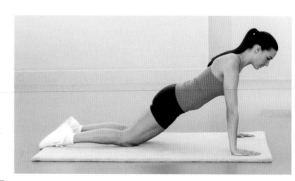

Upper body   *Half Push-up*
Inhale as you bend your elbows, lowering your chest to the floor. Exhale as you push up to the starting position. Count how many you can do consecutively without a rest.

Your score

Excellent	20 reps or more
Good	15–19 reps
Fair	10–14 reps
Poor	10 reps or less

PAR-Q AND YOU A questionnaire for people aged 15 to 69 Physical Activity Readiness Questionnaire – PAR-Q (revised 2002)

Regular physical activity is fun and healthy, and increasingly more people are starting to become more active every day. Being more active is perfectly safe for most people. However, some people should check with their doctor before they start becoming much more physically active than they are already.

If you are planning to become much more physically active than you are now, start by answering the seven questions in the box below. If you are between the ages of 15 and 69, the PAR-Q will tell you if you should check with your doctor before you start. If you are over 69 years of age, and you are not used to being very active, check with your doctor.

Common sense is your best guide when you answer these questions. Please read the questions carefully and answer each one honestly: check YES or NO.

YES NO

☐ ☐ **1** Has your doctor ever said that you have a heart condition <u>and</u> that you should only do physical activity recommended by a doctor?

☐ ☐ **2** Do you feel pain in your chest when you do physical activity?

☐ ☐ **3** In the past month, have you had chest pain when you were not doing physical activity?

☐ ☐ **4** Do you lose your balance because of dizziness or do you ever lose consciousness?

YES NO

☐ ☐ **5** Do you have a bone or joint problem (for example, back, knee, or hip) that could possibly be made worse by a marked change in your physical activity?

☐ ☐ **6** Is your doctor currently prescribing drugs (for example, water pills) for your blood pressure or heart condition?

☐ ☐ **7** Do you know of any other reason why you should not do physical activity?

If you answered YES to one or more questions

Talk with your doctor by phone or in person BEFORE you start becoming much more physically active or BEFORE you have a fitness appraisal.
Tell your doctor about the PAR-Q and which questions you answered YES.
• You may be able to do any activity you want – as long as you start slowly and build up gradually. Or, you may need to restrict your activities to those which are safe for you. Talk with your doctor about the kinds of activities you wish to participate in and follow his/her advice.
• Find out which community programmes are going to prove safe and helpful for you.

If you answered NO to all questions

If you answered NO honestly to all PAR-Q questions, you can be reasonably sure that you can:
• start becoming much more physically active – begin slowly and build up gradually. This is the safest and easiest way to go.
• take part in a fitness appraisal – this is an excellent way to determine your basic fitness so that you can plan the best way for you to live actively. It is also highly recommended that you have your blood pressure evaluated. If your reading is over 144/94, talk with your doctor before you start becoming much more physically active.

DELAY BECOMING MUCH MORE ACTIVE:
• if you are not feeling well because of a temporary illness such as a cold or a fever – wait until you feel better
• if you are or may be pregnant – talk to your doctor before you start becoming more active.

PLEASE NOTE:
If your health changes so that you then answer YES to any of the above questions, tell your fitness or health professional. Ask whether you should change your physical activity plan.

Source: Physical Activity Readiness Questionnaire (PAR-Q) © 2002. Reprinted by permission from the Canadian Society for Exercise Physiology. http://www.csep.ca/forms.asp

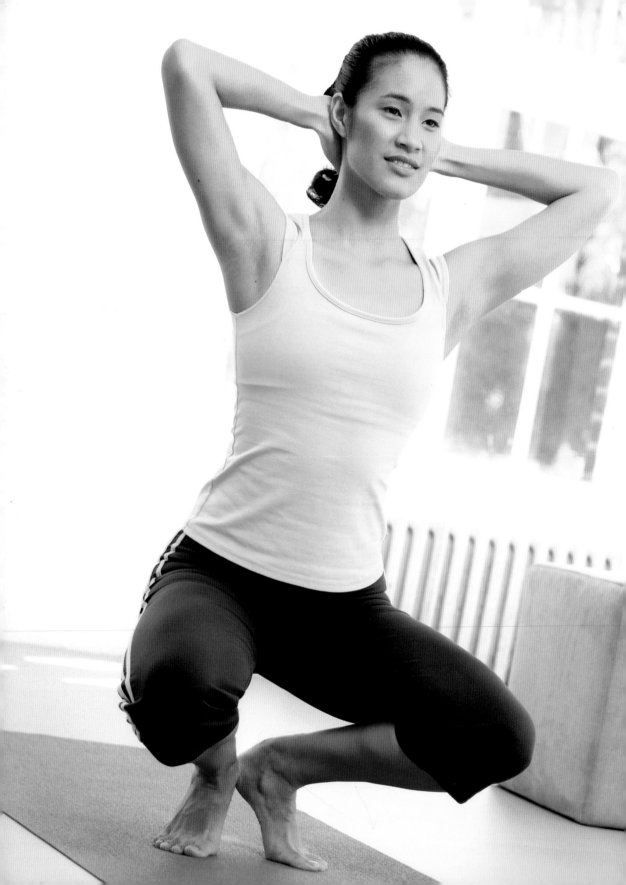

>> **15**minute

everyday
pilates

Alycea Ungaro P.T.

>> **what you need** to start

People spend so much time getting ready to exercise that many never actually do it. I have a badge that reads, "I'm in no shape to exercise".This is an unfortunate and all-too common sentiment. Contrary to popular belief, it is unnecessary to prepare for exercise. You simply must decide to begin.

You will need nothing more than some 1kg (2lb) hand weights and a well-padded mat. Since some rolling exercises can cause bruising on an unpadded surface, many yoga mats may be unsuitable. Instead, choose a mat specifically for Pilates. Finally, keep a towel handy as well as some water, and you'll be ready to go.

Clothing is next. I once had a client with knock knees who happened to be wearing trousers with a seam down the front of the legs. Without thinking, I asked her to position her legs so that the seam was perfectly straight. Voilà! Her legs were better aligned and most importantly, she could see it herself. Whenever possible, select clothing with stripes or visible seams. You'll immediately notice asymmetries and will naturally correct them.

Pilates is normally performed barefoot. However, studios and health clubs often institute a footwear requirement. Bare feet are fine for the home, but for other settings, look for socks with grips to reduce slippage and protect your feet. There are even socks with compartments for each toe. Whatever you select, be sure to avoid slippery socks or cumbersome shoes that might reduce foot mobility.

Where to work out

The single largest impediment to any exercise programme is inconvenience, so find yourself a

A proper Pilates mat, a hand towel and some small hand weights (1kg/2lb) are all you need to begin these Pilates programmes. Be sure you have a clear space to work out.

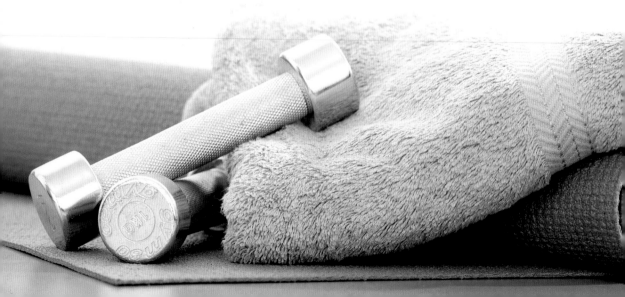

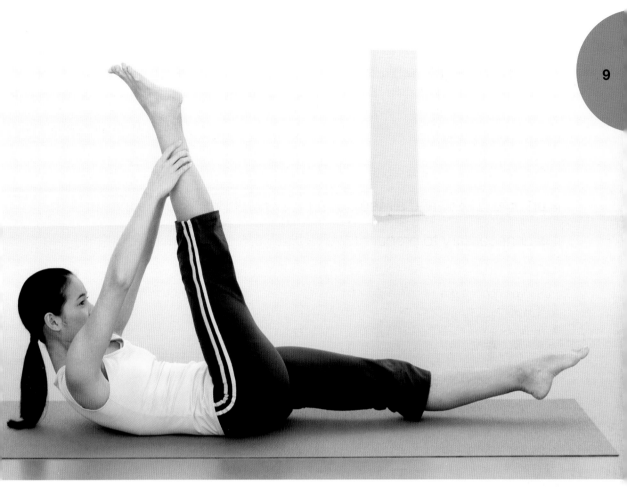

place that is easy to get to and a time that is convenient for your schedule. Pilates can be done anywhere you have enough room to stretch out on a mat. You can practise at a gym or at home. You can even practise on a lawn or beach, as long as you have an appropriate mat.

The safety instinct

Have you ever heard a little voice inside your head cautioning you to stop what you were doing? Did you listen? If you did, you are probably naturally intuitive about safety. For the rest of us, developing that intuition will be largely trial and error. To keep you working out safely, here are some guidelines:

1 Begin with just one programme.

2 Remember to hydrate. By the time you feel thirsty, you are already dehydrated.

3 Learn to distinguish between effort and pain. Effort is OK; pain is a signal to stop.

4 If something doesn't "feel" right, stop.

Clothing can be a visual aid as you work out. Selecting attire with stripes can help you establish good alignment and make improvements to your form.

>> **tips for** getting started

- **Don't waste time** getting ready to exercise. You are ready. Just begin.

- **If a mat is not readily available** use some folded blankets or large towels instead. Plush carpeting can also be a suitable workout surface.

- **Find a time of day** when your energy is at its lowest. Just lying down for one exercise will get your blood flowing and will give you an energy burst.

>> **pilates** from the inside out

Therapists train their patients to become self-aware. This is a significant step towards mental and emotional wellbeing. Similarly, exercise instructors teach you to become physically self-aware. By recognizing your habits and body mechanics, you can embark upon a path of physical health and wellbeing.

Your body is amazing. The coordination of events required for simple actions such as bending your knee or opening your hand is astonishing, yet they happen without us noticing a thing.

By contrast, Pilates teaches your mind to train your body very consciously. During the programmes you will continually be required to recognize your positions, make adjustments and note how you feel. In addition, you must also be focused on the order of exercises, so that you can anticipate and prepare for the next move.

This "mind–body" connection often suggests a workout that is neither physical nor rigorous, but Pilates is both. Just because we think our way through Pilates does not make it less taxing on the muscles. In fact, just the opposite is true. In the words of the late Frederick Schiller, "It is the mind itself that builds the body". Joseph Pilates, the founder of Pilates, was quite fond of this saying.

Learning new patterns

Our brains are built to learn new patterns. As we learn new skills, connections between previously unconnected brain cells are formed. Repetition is key. Each time you do a correct abdominal curl you are building a connection that makes it easier to do correctly the next time. In sum, "cells that fire together, wire together".

Pilates trains this mind-to-body dialogue. You will learn to direct your actions on a gross motor scale as well as a fine motor scale so your results will be amplified and expedited.

>> **just make it** happen

- **Pay attention to your body** throughout your day. Self-awareness is key to good health. If you watch how you move, your exercise routine will improve.

- **Exercise is an activity.** It is not something that happens to you – you make it happen.

- **It requires more energy to avoid** something than simply to do it. Don't waste any time making excuses. Just hit the mat and get started!

Your Pilates body

As you read this book and progress through the workouts, you will find instructions for and mentions of specific parts of your body. The chart opposite is a handy reference guide to them. For ease of use, we have chosen lay-person terms rather than anatomical ones. Names and labels allow your mind to grasp more effectively what is required of you, so become familiar with them and use them as you move through your workout. Think of the chart as a map for your mind.

Remember these simple names for your body parts. Learning about your anatomy will help you identify trouble spots as well as areas of strength in your body.

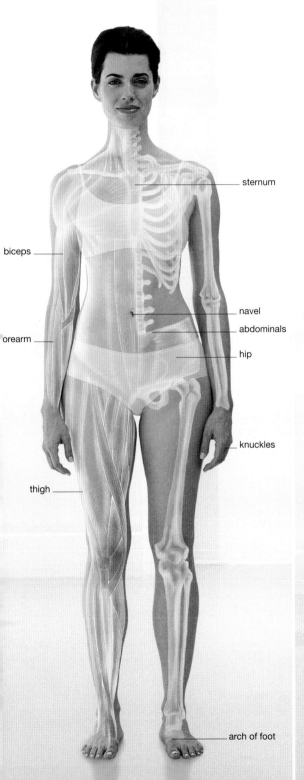

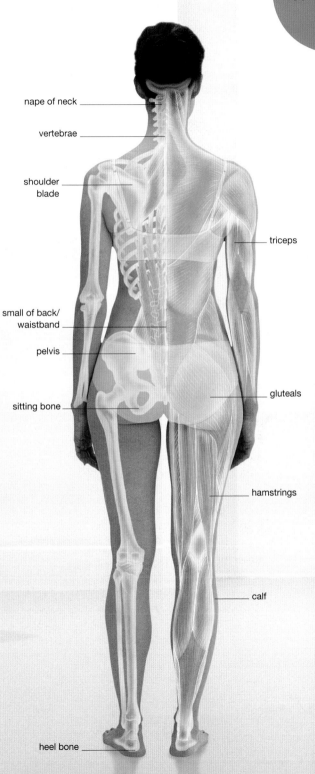

sternum

biceps

navel

abdominals

forearm

hip

knuckles

thigh

arch of foot

nape of neck

vertebrae

shoulder blade

triceps

small of back/ waistband

pelvis

gluteals

sitting bone

hamstrings

calf

heel bone

>> **pilates** concepts

Your Pilates technique and form can constantly be improved upon. Just as musicians must rehearse tirelessly, so Pilates will only get better as you train. Think of it as a language. First you learn the words, then some phrases, and finally you work on your accent. Let's begin here with your first Pilates words.

Before you can start on the mechanics of Pilates, there are six fundamental principles that you should become familiar with. These principles give substance and purpose to the workouts and help you learn to integrate your workout into your life so you begin to feel healthy and strong. Remember, the benefits of Pilates are meant to extend well beyond the actual workout.

Control

This is the primary principle of the system. In his time, Joseph Pilates called his method "Contrology". His focus on controlled movement was a result of his years of blending Eastern and Western disciplines. As you work out, control your muscles, your positions, and your tempos. Your body is your tool and by exerting control over it, it will produce better and better results.

Centring

This is a somewhat vague principle to many people. The idea is that all movement begins from your centre. I'm of the mind that Pilates was really drawing on the principle that you must "stabilize before you mobilize". In Pilates we brace or stabilize the core and then mobilize the limbs. Beyond that, there is an energetic component in working from your centre. It's as though you were able to harness and then project out through the limbs all of the energy and activity going on in your internal organs. Centring is akin to saying you should work from the inside out.

>> **tips for** surefire success

- **Don't over-analyse the work.** Pilates is complicated but it's meant to be a moving system. Keep moving at all costs.

- **Working out is an extension of your life.** Put the same effort into it that you would into anything else.

- **Don't work out – work in!** Inner work shapes the outer body.

- **Never say die.** If an exercise is easy, you're not working hard enough.

- **Don't ask what** an exercise is good for. Mr Pilates said, "It's good for the body."

Concentration

Concentration is key to Pilates. Without focused concentration, any exercise can only be moderately beneficial. Concentration elevates your intensity and so takes your results up to a far higher level.

Precision

This is the fourth principle and just as many of the other principles apply globally, so "precision" serves as an umbrella for this whole list. Attention to the smallest detail is what makes Pilates so effective.

Breath

Breathing is a focus of the Pilates work. Many people come to Pilates because they have heard that it is a breathing technique. You will learn step-by-step breathing in these programmes but it is not their focus. As a general rule, inhale to prepare for a movement and exhale as you execute it.

Flow of movement

This is an element that comes later in the practice but can be incorporated early on. As you learn each exercise, be sure to perform it in a seamless, flowing manner. Eventually you'll work on creating one long routine.

Minimum of movement

Other ideas and concepts, such as symmetry, balance, and integration arise as instructors make their own contributions to Pilates. All of these are applicable but Mr Pilates clearly intended his work to be succinct, so when establishing its main tenets, he chose only the key moves and critical concepts. This working list of six incorporates all the dozens of ideas and concepts at play in Pilates.

Off the floor and out the door

Now that you've learned the six principles, think about how they apply to real life. Concepts such as control, precision or breath can be applied to your life anywhere and anytime. Your workout should be a microcosm of how you live. If you never did any of these programmes, you could still embark upon a brand-new lifestyle simply by incorporating these key principles.

Working out on your own should be just as focused as working with a trainer. Learn to be your own teacher by cueing and correcting yourself constantly.

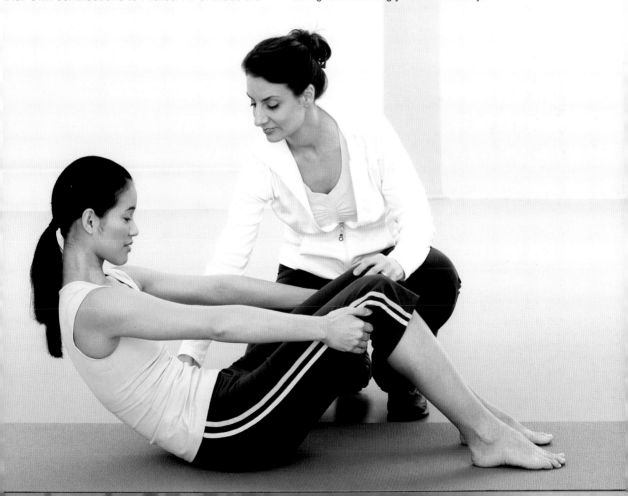

>> **pilates** top to tail

Now that we've covered the ideology of Pilates and the approach you will need to be successful, let's review the physical principles that are present throughout the programmes in this series. Certain elements of positioning are specific to Pilates. Let's start at the top of the body and work our way down.

To keep your neck well aligned during abdominal work, imagine resting your head on a raised support. The curve should be long and natural both front and back. Avoid any crunching or tightening around the throat.

Your breathing in Pilates needs to be specific. The abdominals must work in a contracted fashion at all times so your breathing must be redirected both upwards and outwards. Be aware that your lungs actually extend all the way above your collarbones. Practise breathing laterally, expanding the rib cage sideways as you inhale, and then contracting it inwards as you exhale.

Below the waist

Pilates teachers have several labels for the abdominals, including the core, the centre, and frequently, the powerhouse. No matter the tag,

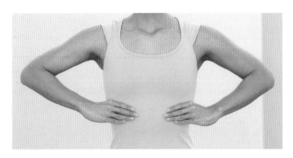

Practise breathing laterally with the hands on either side of the rib cage. On an inhale, the hands should pull apart.

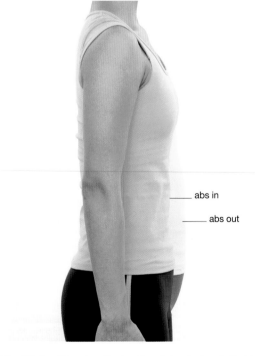

abs in

abs out

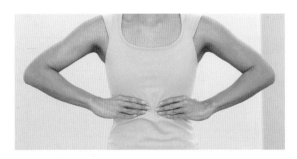

Exhale and feel the ribs narrowing. The hands draw together. Keep the abdominals tight.

The Pilates Scoop activates the abdominal wall. Keep your waist lifted and narrowed. Never allow it to collapse.

your strength and control always spring from the centre of your torso. Your powerhouse specifically incorporates your abs, hips and buttocks as well.

The Pilates Scoop is the signature of the method. Even if you have difficulty pulling the abdominals inwards, you must never allow them to push outwards.

Optimal spinal alignment means positioning your spine to preserve its natural curves. To do this, when you are lying flat for abdominal exercises, try not to tuck or curl the lower back. Instead, aim to lengthen the spine. The end result should be strong, supportive abdominal muscles.

Additionally, when you are working your seat muscles or gluteals, think of "wrapping" the muscles of the buttocks and thighs around towards the back. This will create a tightening and lifting of those muscles and will help to support your spine.

Pilates position or Pilates stance doesn't happen in the feet, although it looks as if it does. Working from your hips down, the gluteal muscles in your rearend and in the backs of your thighs work together to rotate and wrap around. This causes a slight opening of the toes.

Perfect the details

As you work out, focus on your symmetry. Imagine your torso in a box from shoulders to hips. If your box is square, you are probably well aligned. You also need to work within your "frame", which means keeping your limbs within your peripheral vision and never going beyond a comfortable joint range.

Never forget that Pilates is strength training. To maximize its benefits you must always work with resistance. Some resistance is provided by gravity and your positions. More important is the internal resistance you create. Your entire Pilates routine should incorporate this internal resistance.

Opposition is a final but vital ingredient of your Pilates practice. For every action there is an equal and opposite reaction. Pilates is the same. As one side reaches, another side contracts. If you lift up, you also anchor down. By using direct opposition you will find the stability and strength in your core to build a better body.

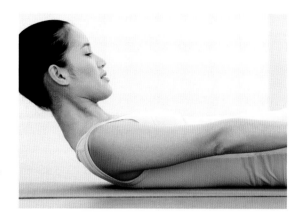

In abdominal work keep your neck lengthened and aligned. Don't force the chin down or tense the throat. Lifting the head comes from your abdominal strength.

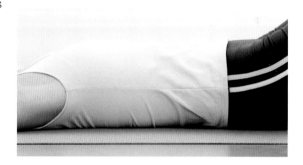

Performing exercises on your back can be tricky for your spine. When working your abdominals, keep your spine lengthened rather than curling it up underneath you.

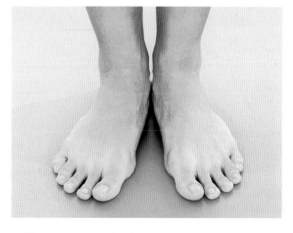

In Pilates stance the heels connect as the toes open. This is achieved by activating and rotating the buttock muscles and the muscles in the backs of the thighs.

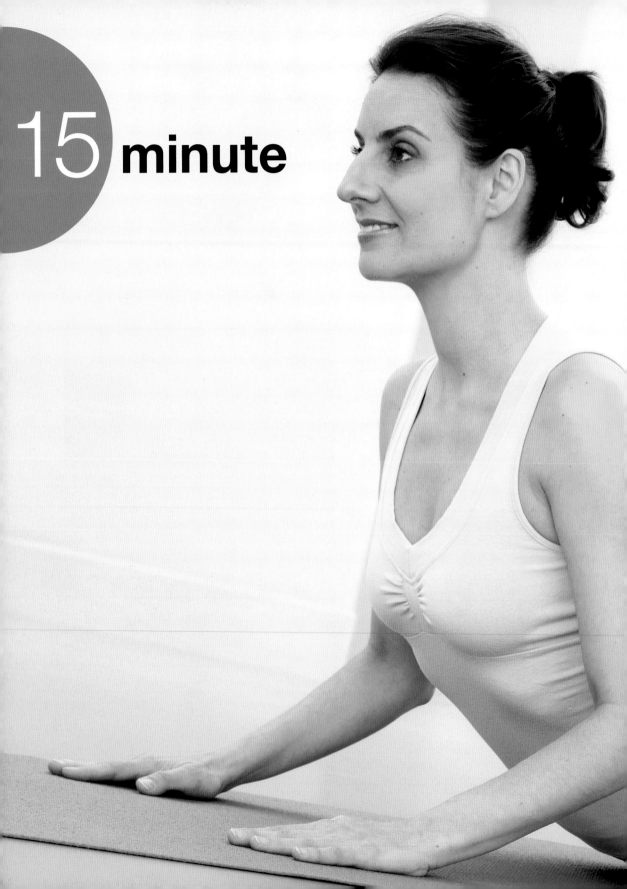

15 minute

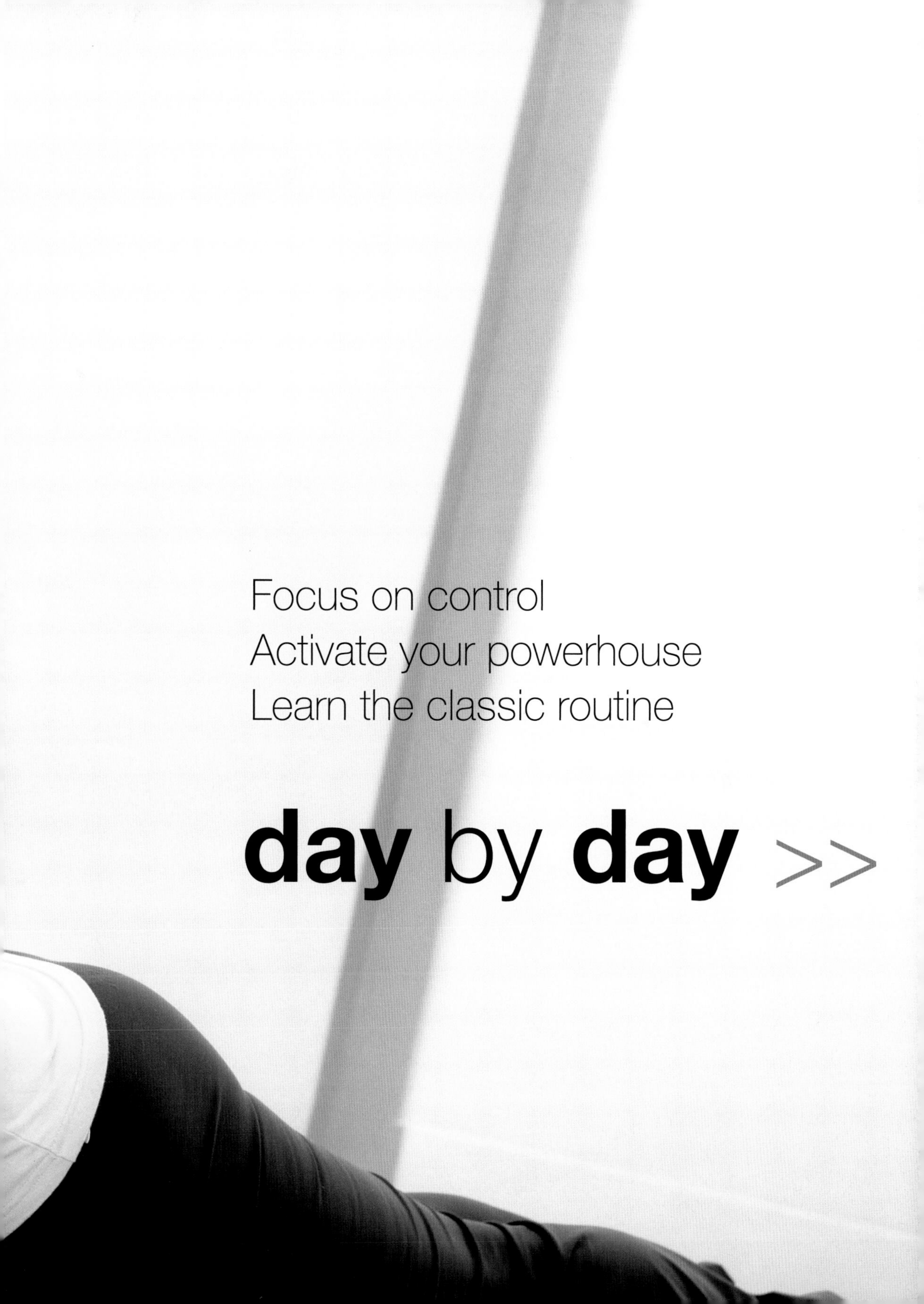

Focus on control
Activate your powerhouse
Learn the classic routine

day by **day** >>

>> abs wake-up

1a Lie flat with your knees bent and your hands across your abs. Even lying flat, your posture should be perfect. Keep your neck long, your shoulders down and your "box" square (see p15). Inhale deeply and let your abs expand. Your hands will lift as you do this.

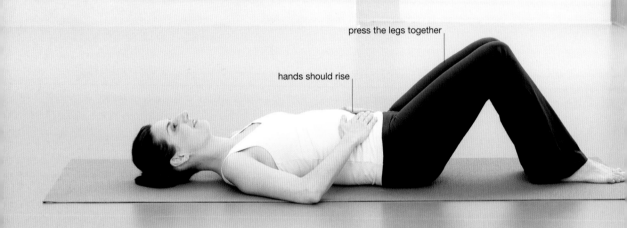

press the legs together

hands should rise

1b Now exhale completely, emptying your lungs and sinking your abs. Don't crunch your midsection or hunch your shoulders. Just pull your belly in deeper, allowing your waist to hollow out. Repeat for 4 repetitions, exhaling longer and contracting deeper with each repetition.

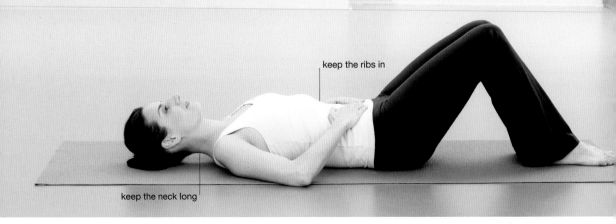

keep the ribs in

keep the neck long

2a

Extend your arms forwards so they hover just above the mat. Your feet remain firmly planted on the mat and your legs are pressed together. Your abs pull inwards and upwards. Prepare to curl up by inhaling.

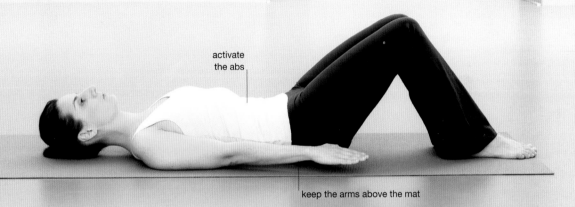

activate the abs

keep the arms above the mat

2b

Exhale, and without letting your abdominal wall expand, lift your head, neck, and shoulders, curling up off the mat. Reach your arms longer and keep focused on your midsection. Lower down smoothly with an inhale. As you repeat, pull in your abs even further. Repeat 3 more times for a total of 4 repetitions.

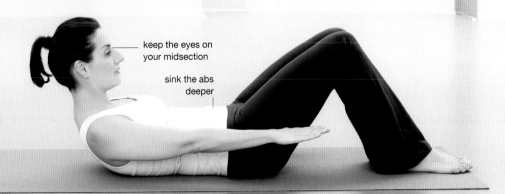

keep the eyes on your midsection

sink the abs deeper

>> the hundred

3a
Begin with both knees drawn into your chest. Curl your upper body up off the mat and reach your arms along your sides just above the mat. Pull in your abs.

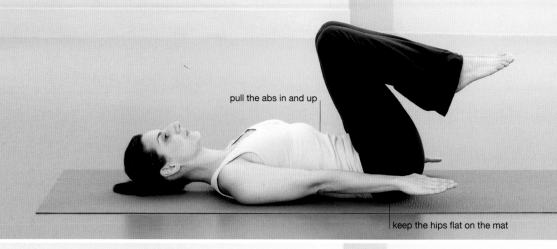

pull the abs in and up

keep the hips flat on the mat

3b
Take both legs up to a 90-degree angle, with your shins parallel to the floor. Pump your arms up and down vigorously, breathing in for 5 pumps and out for 5 pumps. Continue until you reach 100, resting briefly if needed. Keep your abs deep and your torso still and strong.

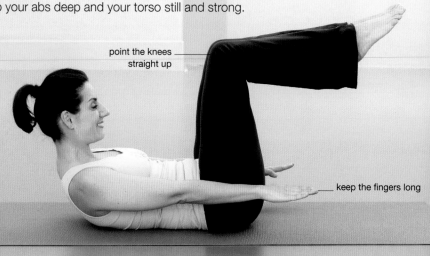

point the knees straight up

keep the fingers long

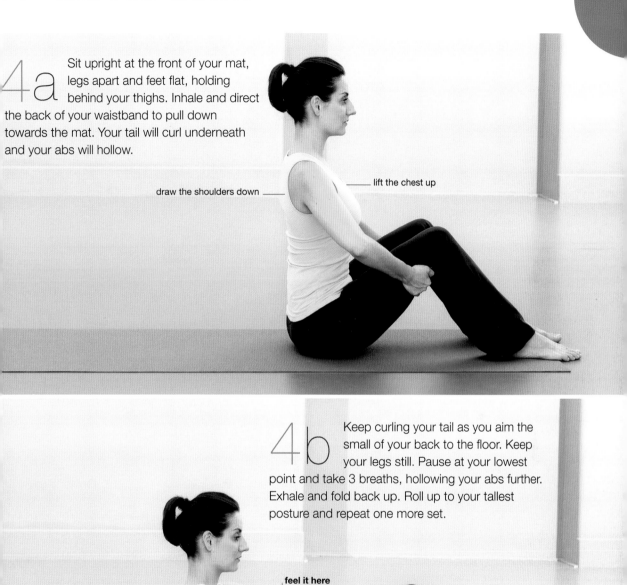

4a Sit upright at the front of your mat, legs apart and feet flat, holding behind your thighs. Inhale and direct the back of your waistband to pull down towards the mat. Your tail will curl underneath and your abs will hollow.

draw the shoulders down _____   _____ lift the chest up

4b Keep curling your tail as you aim the small of your back to the floor. Keep your legs still. Pause at your lowest point and take 3 breaths, hollowing your abs further. Exhale and fold back up. Roll up to your tallest posture and repeat one more set.

feel it here

fold in the waist

>> **single-leg circles**

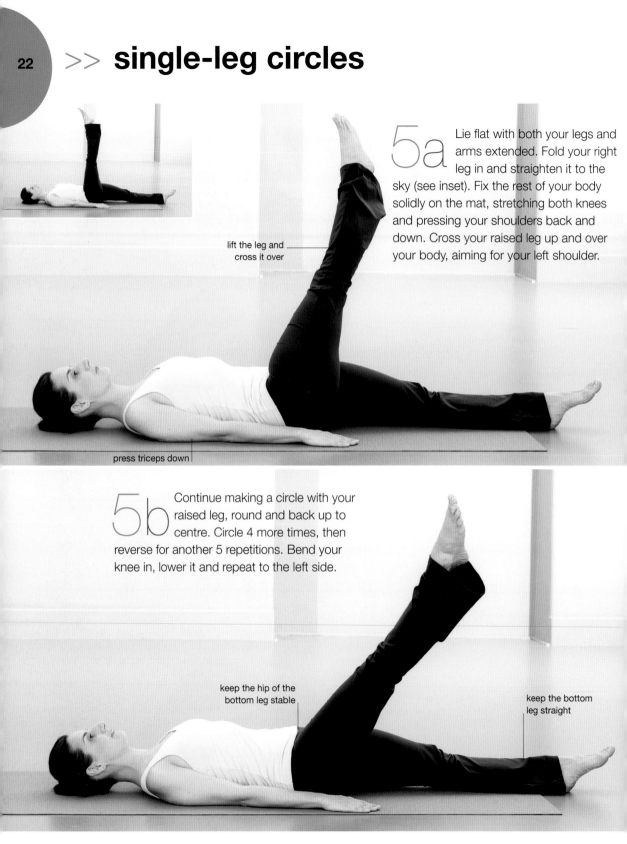

5a Lie flat with both your legs and arms extended. Fold your right leg in and straighten it to the sky (see inset). Fix the rest of your body solidly on the mat, stretching both knees and pressing your shoulders back and down. Cross your raised leg up and over your body, aiming for your left shoulder.

lift the leg and cross it over

press triceps down

5b Continue making a circle with your raised leg, round and back up to centre. Circle 4 more times, then reverse for another 5 repetitions. Bend your knee in, lower it and repeat to the left side.

keep the hip of the bottom leg stable

keep the bottom leg straight

6a Sit at the front edge of your mat, holding behind your thighs with your legs in the air. Keep your shins parallel to the floor. Hold your chest high and scoop your abs. Your elbows are open wide and your ankles are long.

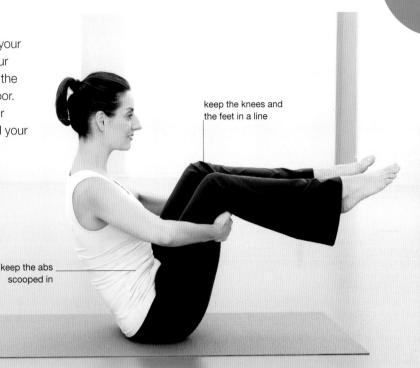

keep the knees and the feet in a line

keep the abs scooped in

6b Tip your pelvis under you, then use your abs to ease back further. At your limit, pull your abs in further and fold your waist, rounding forwards. Sit tall and repeat 3 more times. Lower your feet only after the last repetition.

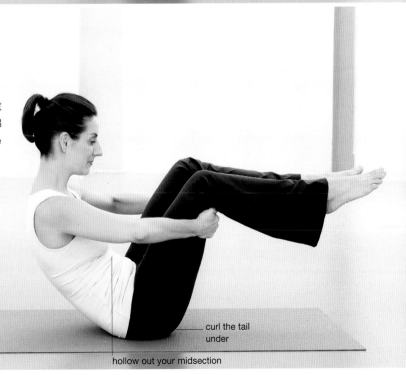

curl the tail under

hollow out your midsection

>> single-leg stretch

7a Lie flat with both knees bent into your chest. Before you curl up, be sure your box or frame is square and then activate your powerhouse (see p15).

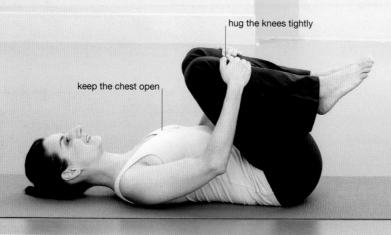

hug the knees tightly

keep the chest open

7b Curl your upper body off the mat and hold your left leg, reaching your left hand to your ankle and the other to your knee. Extend your right leg 45 degrees. Control your torso as you switch legs, inhaling on one side and exhaling on the other. Continue switching for 8 repetitions. Bend both knees to finish. Rest your head.

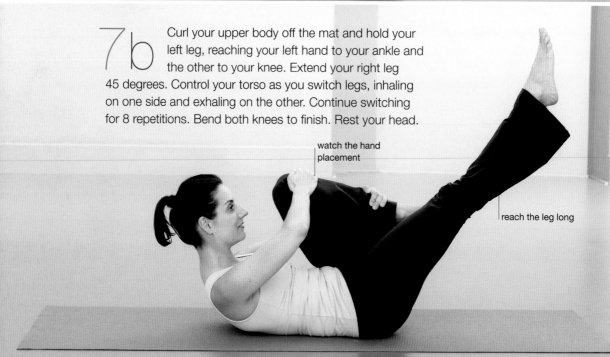

watch the hand placement

reach the leg long

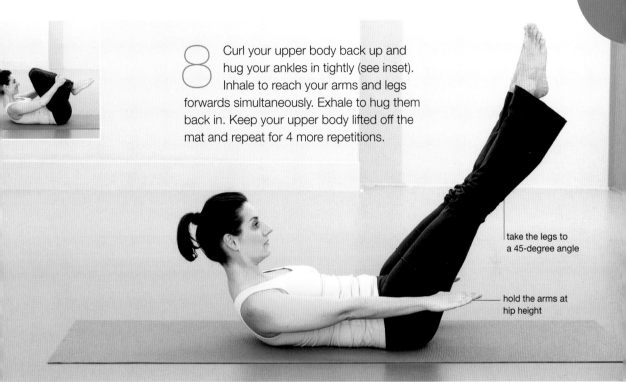

8 Curl your upper body back up and hug your ankles in tightly (see inset). Inhale to reach your arms and legs forwards simultaneously. Exhale to hug them back in. Keep your upper body lifted off the mat and repeat for 4 more repetitions.

take the legs to a 45-degree angle

hold the arms at hip height

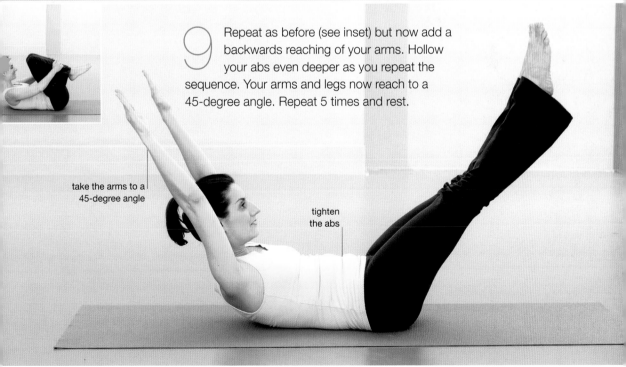

9 Repeat as before (see inset) but now add a backwards reaching of your arms. Hollow your abs even deeper as you repeat the sequence. Your arms and legs now reach to a 45-degree angle. Repeat 5 times and rest.

take the arms to a 45-degree angle

tighten the abs

>> spine stretch forward

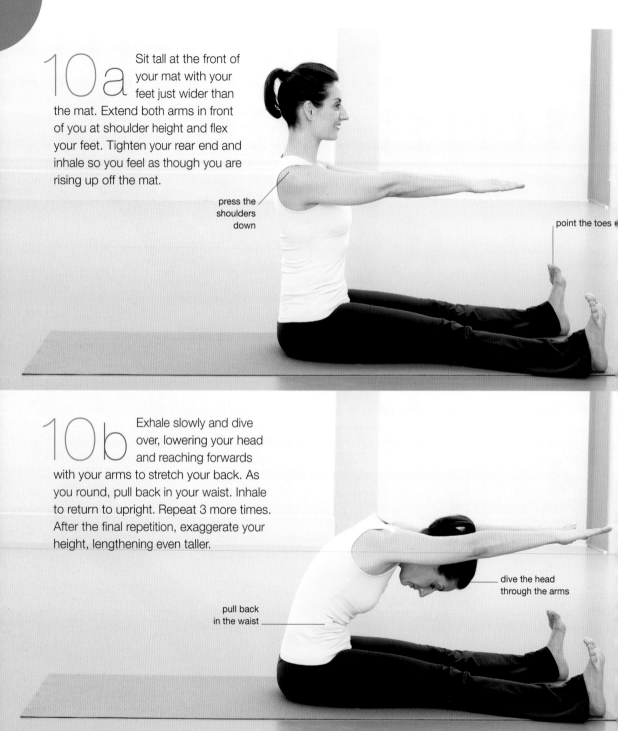

10a Sit tall at the front of your mat with your feet just wider than the mat. Extend both arms in front of you at shoulder height and flex your feet. Tighten your rear end and inhale so you feel as though you are rising up off the mat.

press the shoulders down

point the toes

10b Exhale slowly and dive over, lowering your head and reaching forwards with your arms to stretch your back. As you round, pull back in your waist. Inhale to return to upright. Repeat 3 more times. After the final repetition, exaggerate your height, lengthening even taller.

dive the head through the arms

pull back in the waist

>> the swan/neck roll

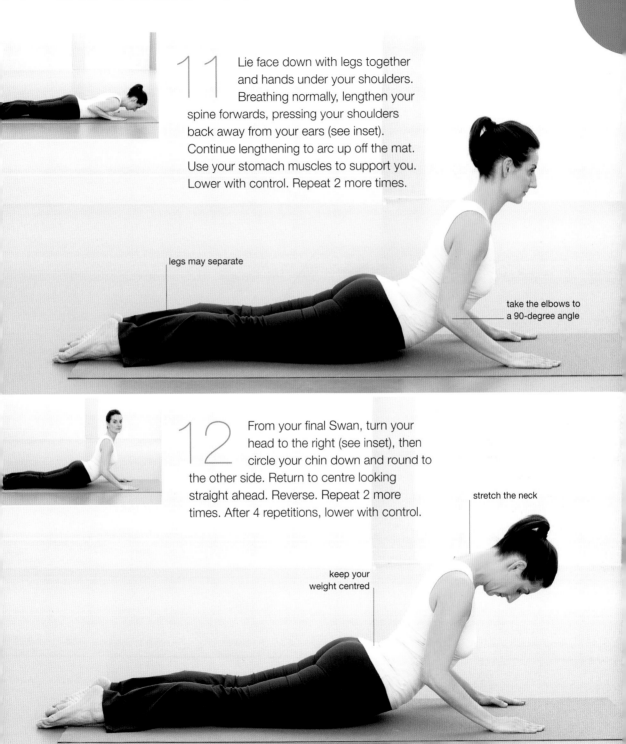

11 Lie face down with legs together and hands under your shoulders. Breathing normally, lengthen your spine forwards, pressing your shoulders back away from your ears (see inset). Continue lengthening to arc up off the mat. Use your stomach muscles to support you. Lower with control. Repeat 2 more times.

legs may separate

take the elbows to a 90-degree angle

12 From your final Swan, turn your head to the right (see inset), then circle your chin down and round to the other side. Return to centre looking straight ahead. Reverse. Repeat 2 more times. After 4 repetitions, lower with control.

stretch the neck

keep your weight centred

>> child's pose/pelvic lift

13 Push back to sit on your heels with your back rounded, hands in front of you. Open your knees slightly to allow your upper body to sink deeper. Keep your abs lifted as you take 3 deep breaths. With each inhale, try to stretch and release your lower-back muscles. With each exhale, draw your navel even higher upwards. After 3 deep breaths, roll up to a kneeling position.

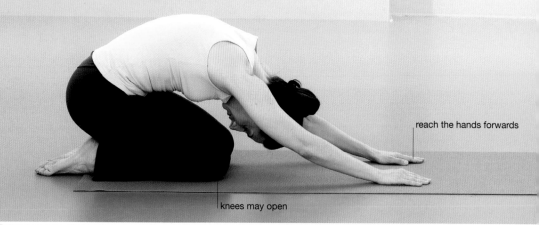

reach the hands forwards

knees may open

14 Lie with knees bent and legs hip-width apart. Feel your chest open, shoulders back and spine long (see inset). Inhale and raise your hips without arching your back. Exhale and lower down, one vertebra at a time. Repeat 3 more times, increasing the articulation of your spine each time.

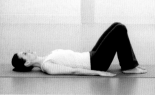

feel it here

reach the knees forwa

keep the ribs in

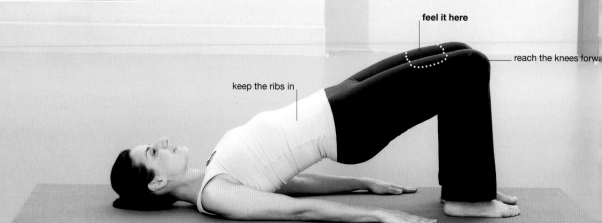

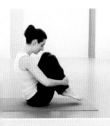

15a

Balance on your sitting bones at the front edge of your mat, hugging your ankles into your body and nestling your head between your knees (see inset). Without letting your feet touch down, tuck your tail under you and begin to roll back.

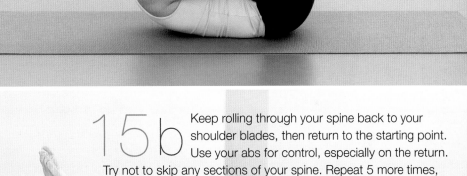

hold the ankles snugly

keep the head tucked in

15b

Keep rolling through your spine back to your shoulder blades, then return to the starting point. Use your abs for control, especially on the return. Try not to skip any sections of your spine. Repeat 5 more times, inhaling as you roll and exhaling as you return.

take the feet close to the buttocks

aim the sitting bones to the sky

don't rock onto the neck

15 minute

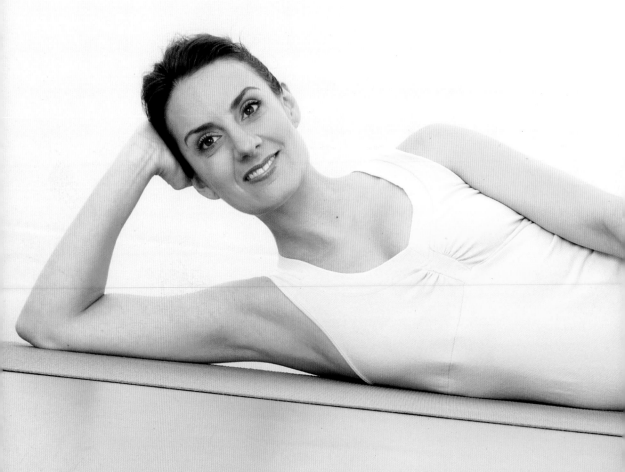

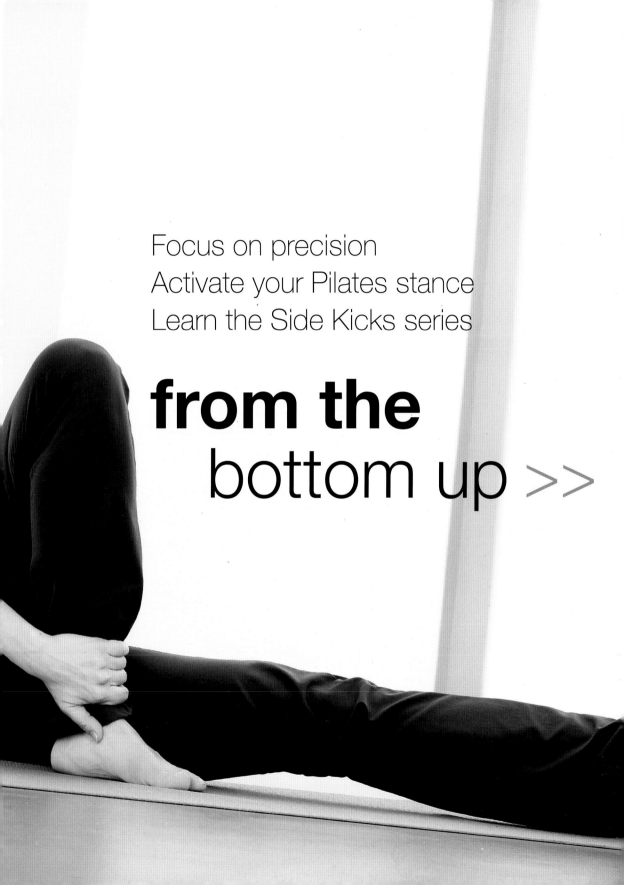

Focus on precision
Activate your Pilates stance
Learn the Side Kicks series

from the
bottom up >>

>> pilates stance 1 and 2

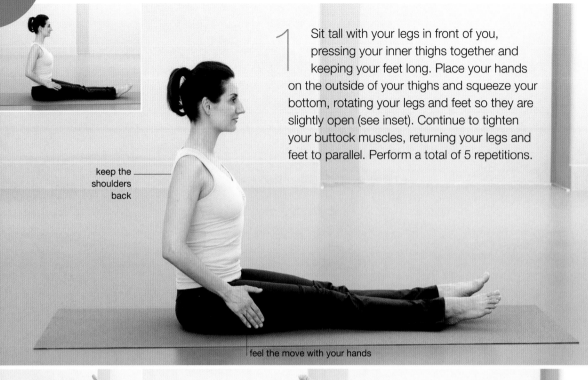

1 Sit tall with your legs in front of you, pressing your inner thighs together and keeping your feet long. Place your hands on the outside of your thighs and squeeze your bottom, rotating your legs and feet so they are slightly open (see inset). Continue to tighten your buttock muscles, returning your legs and feet to parallel. Perform a total of 5 repetitions.

keep the shoulders back

feel the move with your hands

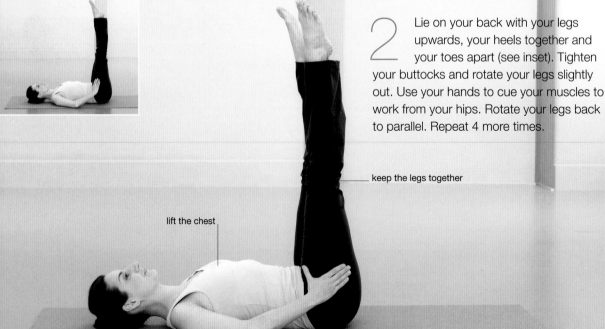

2 Lie on your back with your legs upwards, your heels together and your toes apart (see inset). Tighten your buttocks and rotate your legs slightly out. Use your hands to cue your muscles to work from your hips. Rotate your legs back to parallel. Repeat 4 more times.

keep the legs together

lift the chest

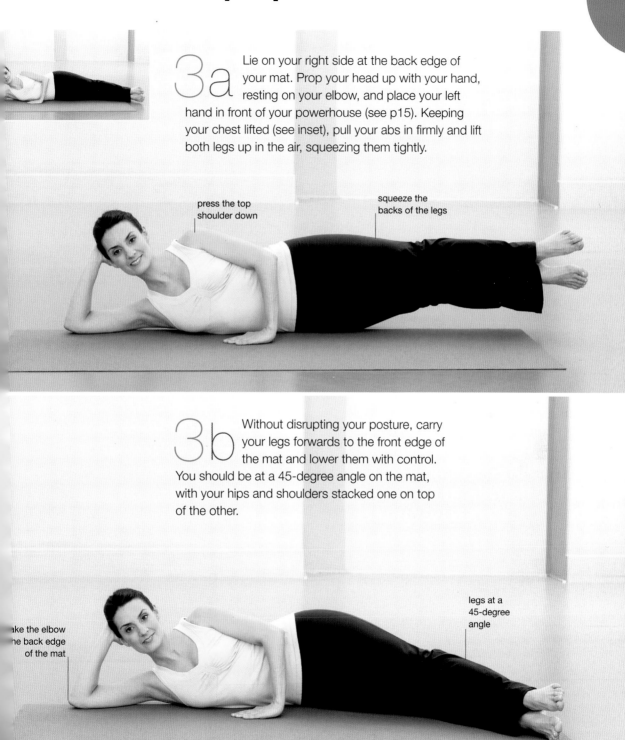

3a
Lie on your right side at the back edge of your mat. Prop your head up with your hand, resting on your elbow, and place your left hand in front of your powerhouse (see p15). Keeping your chest lifted (see inset), pull your abs in firmly and lift both legs up in the air, squeezing them tightly.

press the top shoulder down

squeeze the backs of the legs

3b
Without disrupting your posture, carry your legs forwards to the front edge of the mat and lower them with control. You should be at a 45-degree angle on the mat, with your hips and shoulders stacked one on top of the other.

legs at a 45-degree angle

ake the elbow he back edge of the mat

>> side kicks front

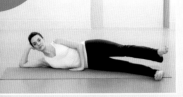

4a Lying on your side at a 45-degree angle on the mat, elevate your left leg and slightly rotate it up to the ceiling. Your right foot remains solidly on the mat, slightly flexed and pressing down into the floor (see inset). Carry your leg forwards in a kicking motion, pulsing twice at the height of your kick.

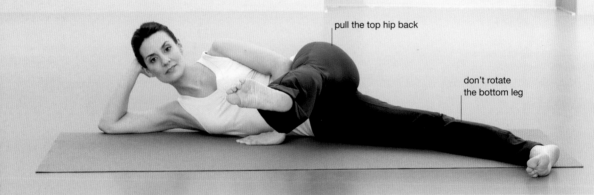

pull the top hip back

don't rotate the bottom leg

4b Sweep your leg down and back behind your body, tightening your buttock muscles. Keep your upper body still and strong. Repeat a total of 6 times, perfecting your form each time. Bring your leg back to its starting position.

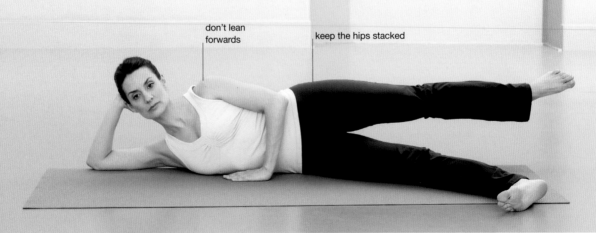

don't lean forwards

keep the hips stacked

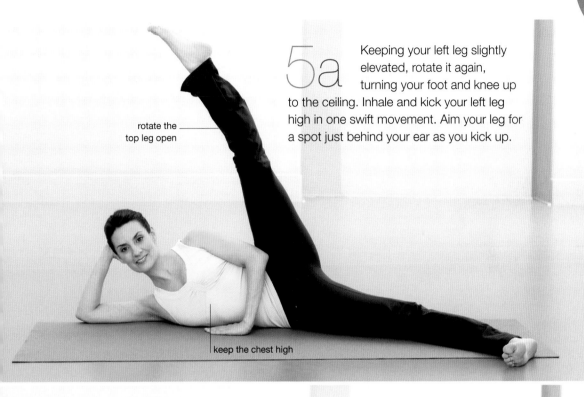

rotate the
top leg open

5a Keeping your left leg slightly elevated, rotate it again, turning your foot and knee up to the ceiling. Inhale and kick your left leg high in one swift movement. Aim your leg for a spot just behind your ear as you kick up.

keep the chest high

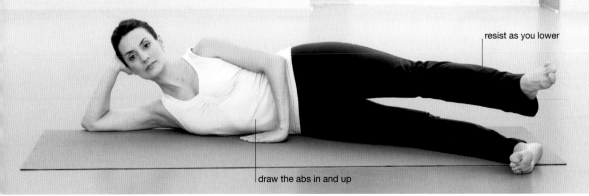

5b Lower your leg down, creating resistance (see p15) as you go, for a count of 3. Use opposition (see p19): as your leg lowers, your abs should draw inwards and upwards. Lift your chest as you repeat 5 more times – for a total of 6 repetitions.

resist as you lower

draw the abs in and up

>> side kicks circles

6a Remain lying on your side. Carry your top leg just in front of your bottom leg. It should feel very heavy at this point. Keep it rotated up to the sky with your ankle long.

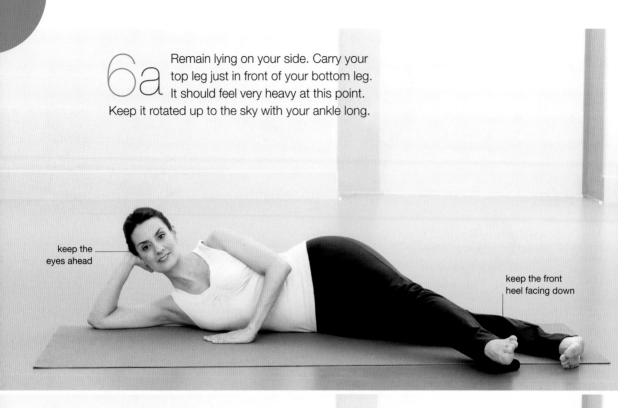

keep the eyes ahead

keep the front heel facing down

6b Draw 10 tiny circles with your leg in the air without shaking your body. Pause briefly. Switch immediately, taking your left leg back and reversing the circles. Keep the circles tiny and emphasize the downwards portion of the circle. Repeat 10 circles and pause before resting your left leg on the right.

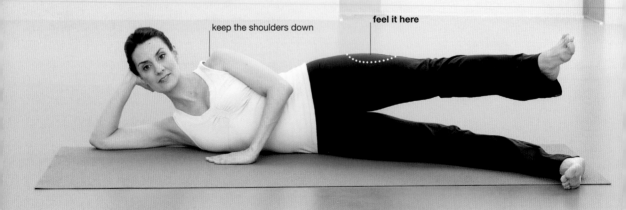

keep the shoulders down

feel it here

>> side kicks inner-thigh lifts

7a Remain lying on your right side. Cross your left leg in front of your right leg and take hold of your ankle. Place your left foot flat on the floor with your knee and foot pointing down towards your bottom foot. Now, flex your right foot and lift your entire right leg just above the mat.

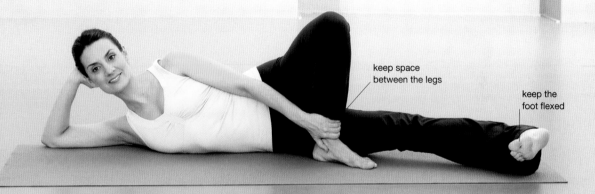

keep space
between the legs

keep the
foot flexed

7b Without hunching or collapsing, raise your right leg to its highest point and lower it back to above the mat. Repeat 7 more times for a total of 8 repetitions. On the last repetition, remain at the highest point and perfect the position by lengthening, straightening and rotating just a little bit more. Finally, lower your leg with control.

keep the chest lifted

foot on the mat angles down

>> side kicks bicycle

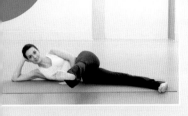

8a

Lie with your legs together at a 45-degree angle in front of you. Raise your left leg slightly. Swing it out in front of your body without hunching or rounding your back (see inset). Create opposition by pulling back, or retracting, your left hip behind you slightly. Bend your left knee in towards your shoulder.

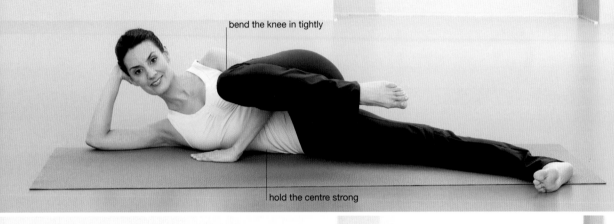

bend the knee in tightly

hold the centre strong

8b

Sweep your left knee down next to your right knee before extending it behind you. Pull your waist up in opposition to your leg reaching down. Repeat 2 more times and then return your leg to its start position. Reverse direction for 3 more repetitions.

reach far behind you

feel it here

tighten the seat

don't lean on the front hand

9a Transition onto your stomach, then lie face down on your mat. Place your hands under your forehead and stretch your legs out. Tighten your abs and elevate both legs slightly. Keep your shoulders pulling back and down as you open your legs and start to beat them together.

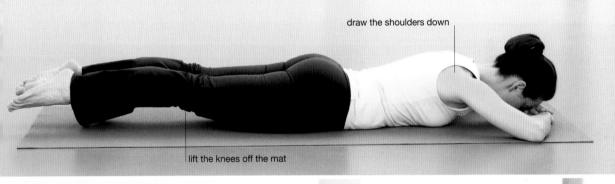

draw the shoulders down

lift the knees off the mat

9b Breathing naturally, continue beating briskly for 20 counts. Beat your legs from your upper inner thighs and keep your knees straight. Pause at the end to lengthen your legs, tighten your abs, and soften your neck and shoulders before lowering your legs with control. Roll over onto the other side and repeat the Side Kicks series (steps 3a–8b) with the opposite leg.

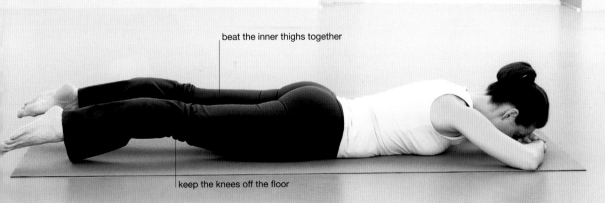

beat the inner thighs together

keep the knees off the floor

>> **the teaser**

10a
Transition onto your back and bring your knees into your chest as you reach your arms overhead.

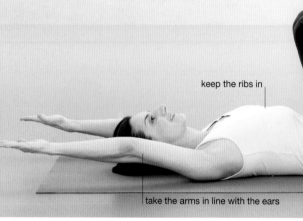

keep the ribs in

take the arms in line with the ears

10b
In one count, sweep your body up to sitting, balancing with your legs at 90 degrees, arms reaching forwards, abs deeply scooped, chest open. With control, curl your tail under you, laying your spine onto the mat. Fold your knees in, arms overhead to repeat. Perform 5 repetitions.

reach beyond the legs

scoop the abs in

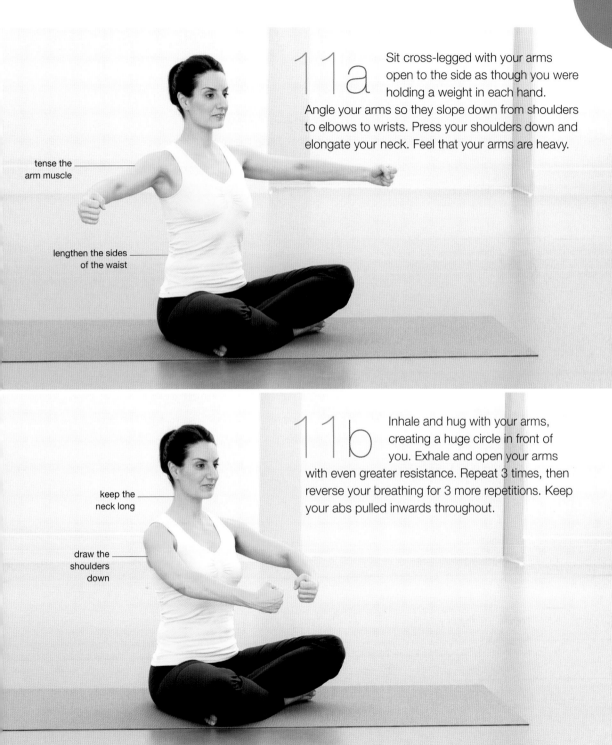

11a

Sit cross-legged with your arms open to the side as though you were holding a weight in each hand. Angle your arms so they slope down from shoulders to elbows to wrists. Press your shoulders down and elongate your neck. Feel that your arms are heavy.

tense the arm muscle

lengthen the sides of the waist

11b

Inhale and hug with your arms, creating a huge circle in front of you. Exhale and open your arms with even greater resistance. Repeat 3 times, then reverse your breathing for 3 more repetitions. Keep your abs pulled inwards throughout.

keep the neck long

draw the shoulders down

>> the mermaid

12a Sit to the right side of your legs with your knees, shins and ankles stacked on your left. Reach your left hand underneath your bottom ankle and hook onto it, holding firmly. Sweep your free right arm up overhead and inhale to prepare.

lengthen the waist _____

hold the bottom
ankle firmly

reach up and over

12b Bend lightly over your legs, exhaling as you stretch your right side. Reach your arm and body higher up as you return to upright. Repeat 2 more times, pausing at the end, lifting your waist and pulling your shoulders down. Swing your legs to the other side for 3 more repetitions.

open the elbow out

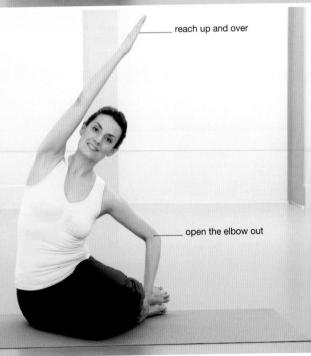

>> arm circles

13a Stand in Pilates stance (see p15). Shift your weight slightly forwards. Hold your arms by your thighs with your palms facing forwards (see inset). Inhale, then exhale and raise your arms straight up to the sky.

13b Flip your palms outwards and circle your arms down, exerting pressure as though the air were thick. Repeat 2 more times, then reverse the breath, inhaling on the raise and exhaling on the lower, for another 3 repetitions.

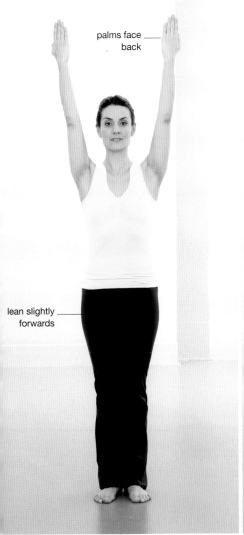

palms face back

lean slightly forwards

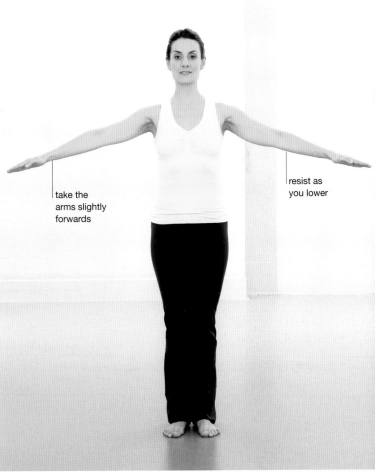

take the arms slightly forwards

resist as you lower

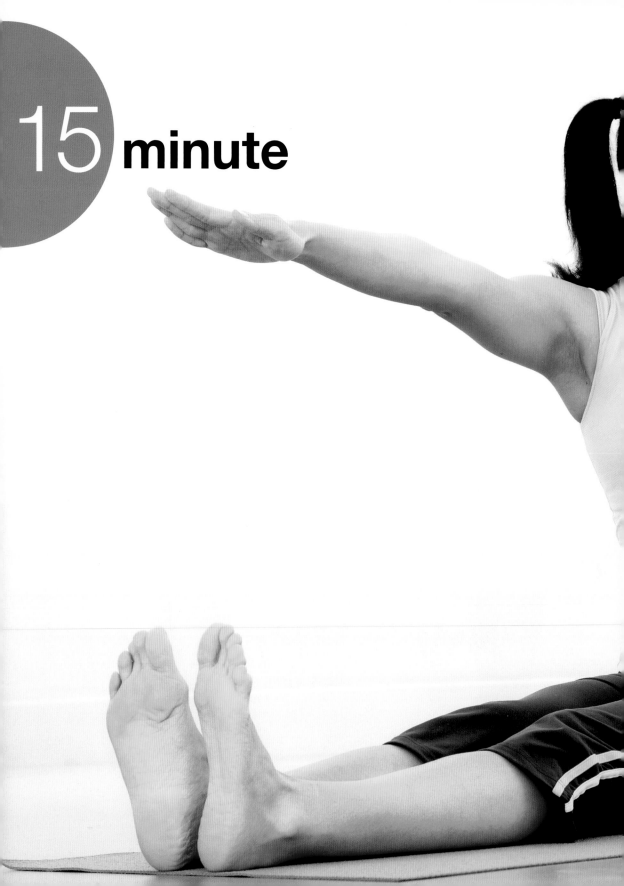

15 minute

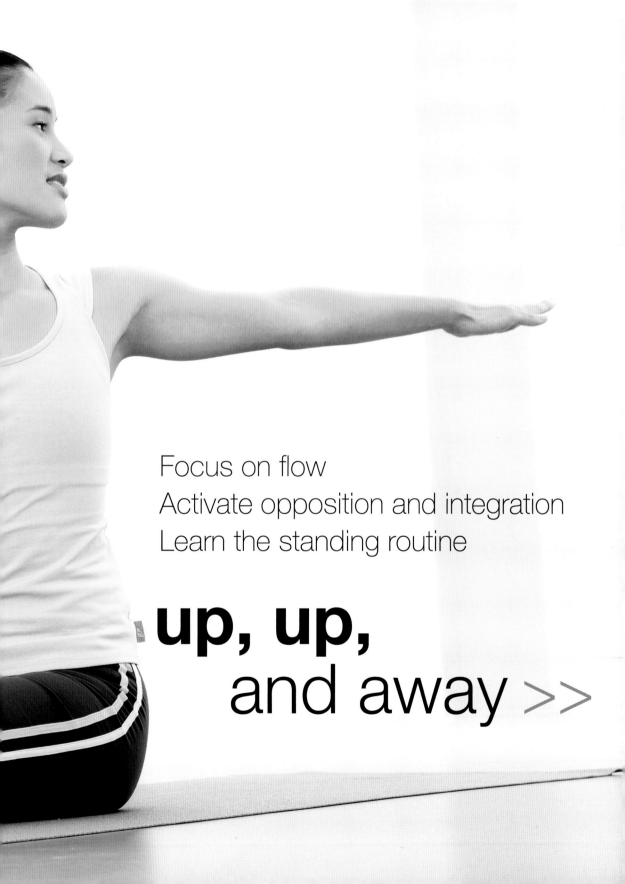

Focus on flow
Activate opposition and integration
Learn the standing routine

up, up, and away >>

>> neck press/shoulder roll

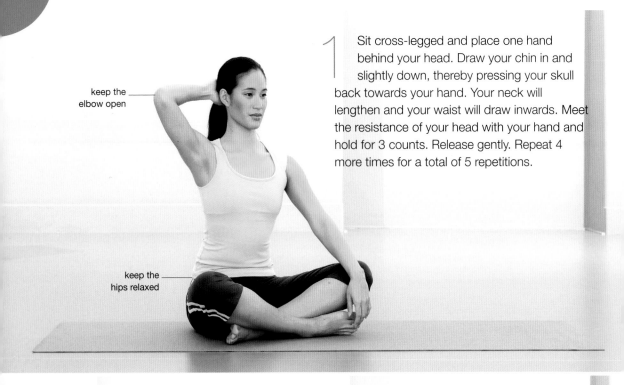

keep the elbow open

keep the hips relaxed

1 Sit cross-legged and place one hand behind your head. Draw your chin in and slightly down, thereby pressing your skull back towards your hand. Your neck will lengthen and your waist will draw inwards. Meet the resistance of your head with your hand and hold for 3 counts. Release gently. Repeat 4 more times for a total of 5 repetitions.

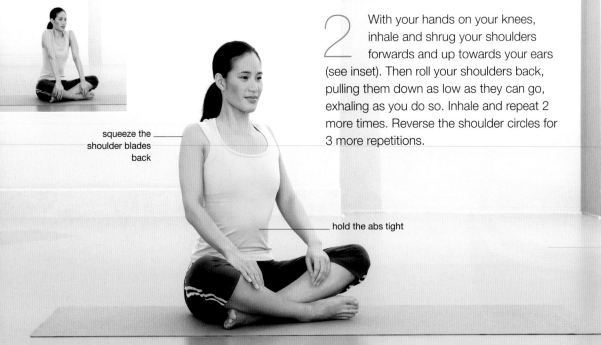

squeeze the shoulder blades back

hold the abs tight

2 With your hands on your knees, inhale and shrug your shoulders forwards and up towards your ears (see inset). Then roll your shoulders back, pulling them down as low as they can go, exhaling as you do so. Inhale and repeat 2 more times. Reverse the shoulder circles for 3 more repetitions.

>> the hundred

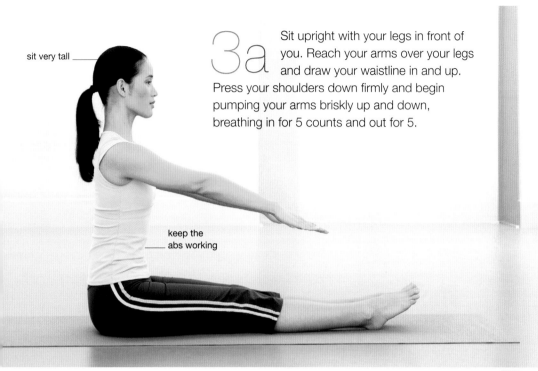

sit very tall

3a

Sit upright with your legs in front of you. Reach your arms over your legs and draw your waistline in and up. Press your shoulders down firmly and begin pumping your arms briskly up and down, breathing in for 5 counts and out for 5.

keep the abs working

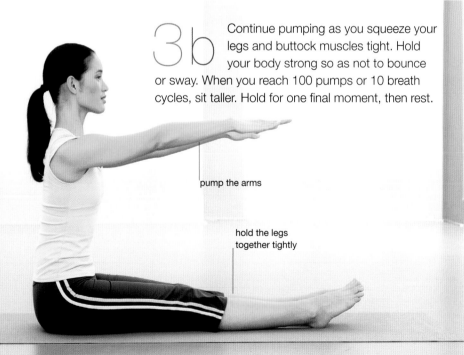

3b

Continue pumping as you squeeze your legs and buttock muscles tight. Hold your body strong so as not to bounce or sway. When you reach 100 pumps or 10 breath cycles, sit taller. Hold for one final moment, then rest.

pump the arms

hold the legs together tightly

>> rowing 1

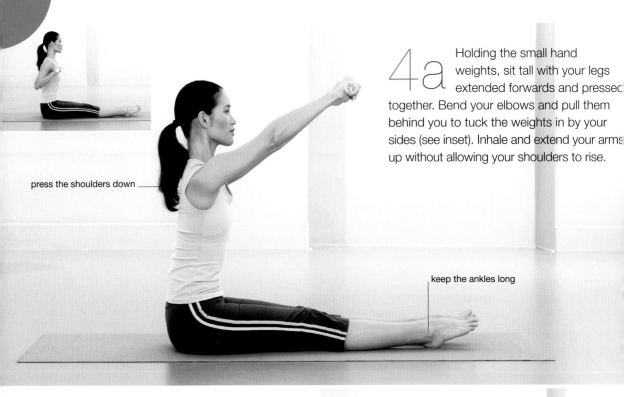

press the shoulders down

keep the ankles long

4a Holding the small hand weights, sit tall with your legs extended forwards and pressed together. Bend your elbows and pull them behind you to tuck the weights in by your sides (see inset). Inhale and extend your arms up without allowing your shoulders to rise.

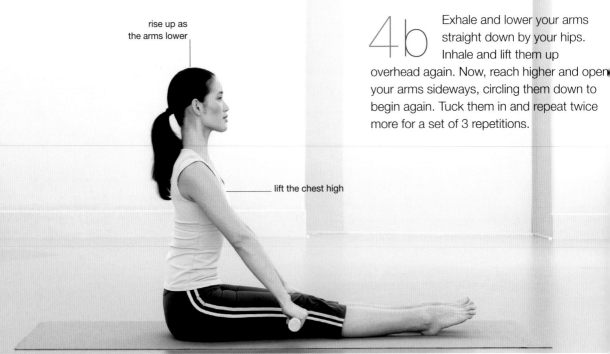

rise up as the arms lower

lift the chest high

4b Exhale and lower your arms straight down by your hips. Inhale and lift them up overhead again. Now, reach higher and open your arms sideways, circling them down to begin again. Tuck them in and repeat twice more for a set of 3 repetitions.

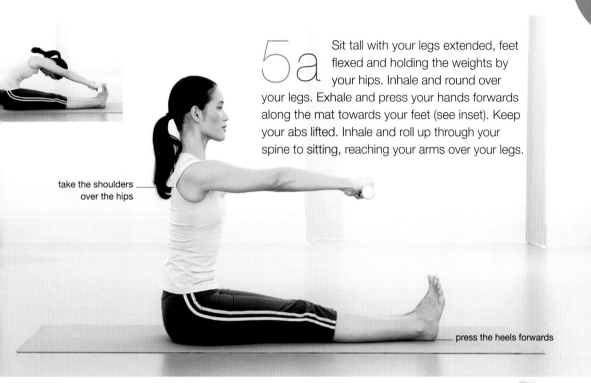

5a
Sit tall with your legs extended, feet flexed and holding the weights by your hips. Inhale and round over your legs. Exhale and press your hands forwards along the mat towards your feet (see inset). Keep your abs lifted. Inhale and roll up through your spine to sitting, reaching your arms over your legs.

take the shoulders over the hips

press the heels forwards

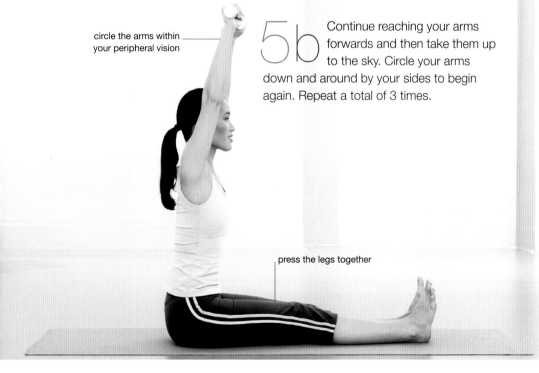

circle the arms within your peripheral vision

5b
Continue reaching your arms forwards and then take them up to the sky. Circle your arms down and around by your sides to begin again. Repeat a total of 3 times.

press the legs together

up, up, and away >>

>> spine twist

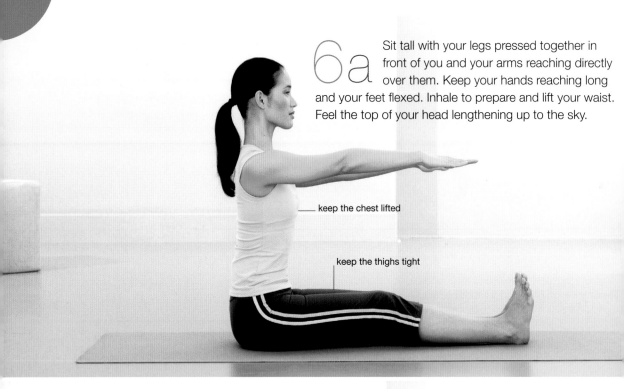

6a Sit tall with your legs pressed together in front of you and your arms reaching directly over them. Keep your hands reaching long and your feet flexed. Inhale to prepare and lift your waist. Feel the top of your head lengthening up to the sky.

— keep the chest lifted

keep the thighs tight

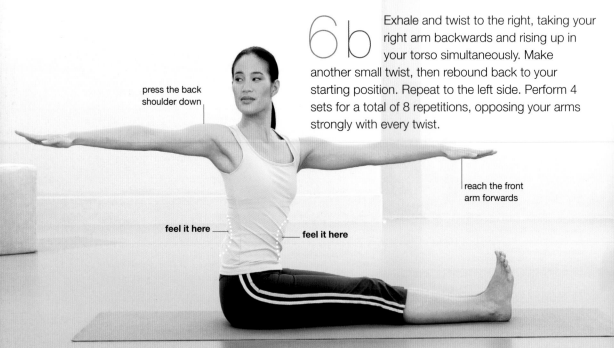

6b Exhale and twist to the right, taking your right arm backwards and rising up in your torso simultaneously. Make another small twist, then rebound back to your starting position. Repeat to the left side. Perform 4 sets for a total of 8 repetitions, opposing your arms strongly with every twist.

press the back
shoulder down

reach the front
arm forwards

feel it here

feel it here

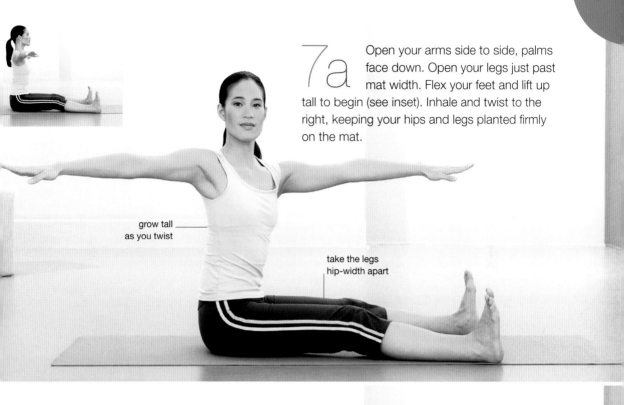

7a Open your arms side to side, palms face down. Open your legs just past mat width. Flex your feet and lift up tall to begin (see inset). Inhale and twist to the right, keeping your hips and legs planted firmly on the mat.

grow tall as you twist

take the legs hip-width apart

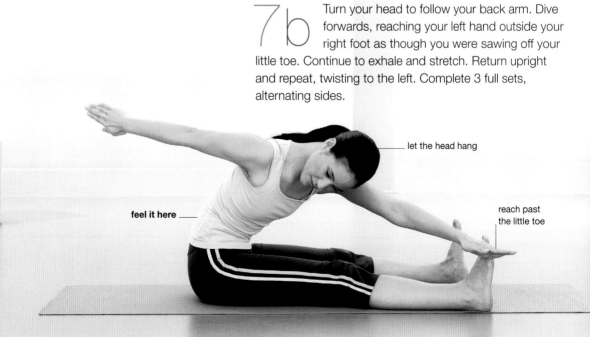

7b Turn your head to follow your back arm. Dive forwards, reaching your left hand outside your right foot as though you were sawing off your little toe. Continue to exhale and stretch. Return upright and repeat, twisting to the left. Complete 3 full sets, alternating sides.

let the head hang

feel it here

reach past the little toe

>> lotus

8a Take your weights and kneel upright on your mat with your knees comfortably apart. Your arms extend to the sides of your body with your palms face up. Hold strong in your core and keep your chest lifted.

8b Without disrupting your posture, raise your arms straight up, framing your head and neck in an oval. Lower your arms back down with controlled resistance (see p15). Keep your elbows soft. Repeat for a total of 8 times, exhaling to lift and inhaling to lower.

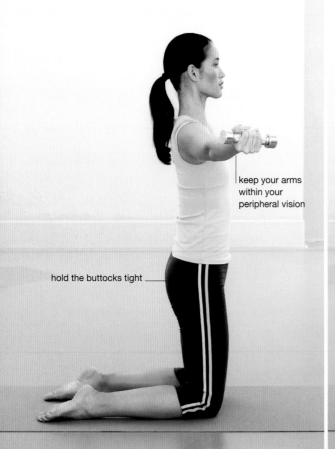

keep your arms within your peripheral vision

hold the buttocks tight

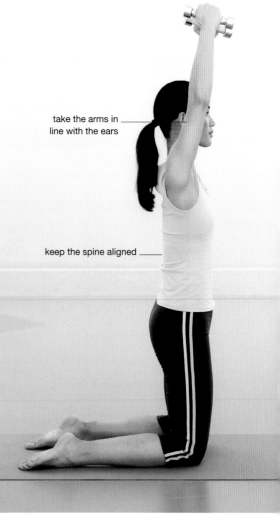

take the arms in line with the ears

keep the spine aligned

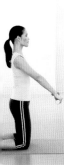

9a Still kneeling upright, hold the weights just in front of you (see inset). Tighten your buttocks and pull up in your waist to activate your core. Inhale and sweep your arms behind you with resistance, opening your chest and drawing your shoulder blades together as you go.

9b Keep your arms behind you as you look over your right shoulder and then the left before returning to centre. Exhale and take your arms back in front of you. Repeat 3 more times, alternating the initial direction you turn your head with each set.

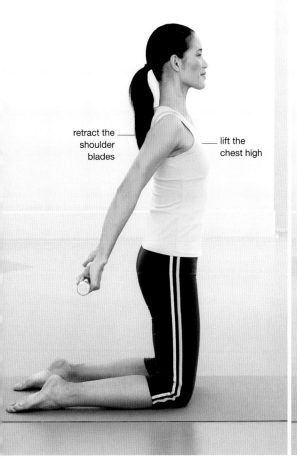

retract the shoulder blades

lift the chest high

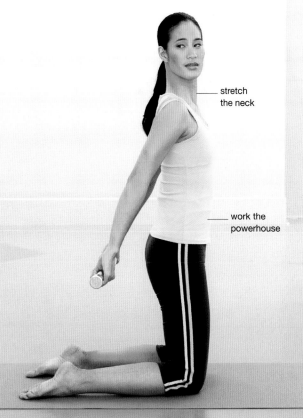

stretch the neck

work the powerhouse

>> thigh stretch

10a Remain on your knees holding the weights with your arms extended directly in front of you just below shoulder height. Face your palms down and tighten your powerhouse (see p15) to begin. Inhale to prepare.

10b Allow your chin to dip down slightly then hinge back, stretching the fronts of your thighs but not arching your spine. At your lowest point, tighten your buttocks and bring your body back up to start again. Perform a total of 4 repetitions, exhaling each time you rise back up. Put the weights down. Tuck your toes under you to come up to standing.

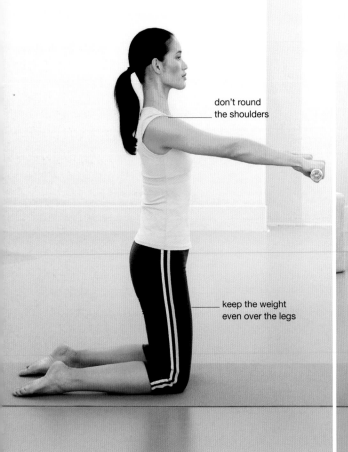

don't round the shoulders

keep the weight even over the legs

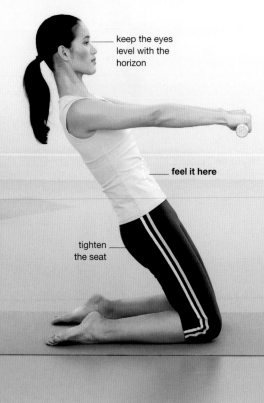

keep the eyes level with the horizon

feel it here

tighten the seat

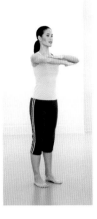

11 Come off your mat and stand up tall in Pilates stance (see p19). Place your hands behind your head, elbows wide (see inset). Inhale and bend your knees to lower into a squat. Allow your heels to rise. At the bottom of the squat, press your heels into the floor to rise back up. Perform 6 times, inhaling to lower and exhaling to rise.

12 Stand with feet parallel, hip-width apart, arms folded in front of you at chest height (see inset). Bend your knees as low as you can go, then push your feet into the floor to rise. Repeat for 6 repetitions. Inhale to lower and exhale to rise.

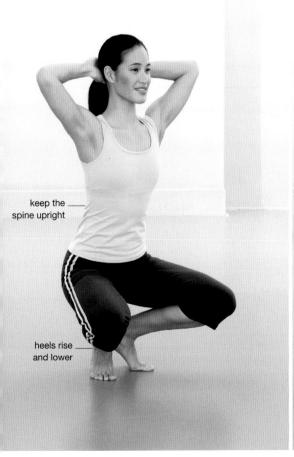

keep the spine upright

heels rise and lower

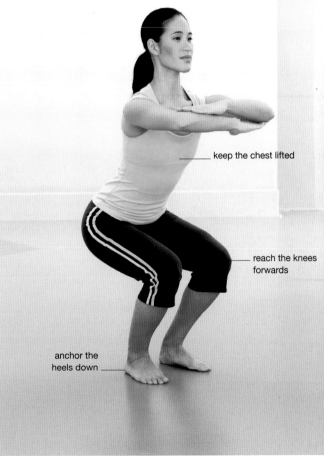

keep the chest lifted

reach the knees forwards

anchor the heels down

>> footwork 3/tendon stretch

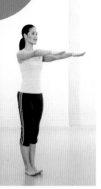

13 Standing with feet together and arms extended in front for stability, curl your toes up and press the rest of your foot firmly down (see inset). Pull your abs in, then bend into a squat. Keep your heels down if possible and stay as upright as you can, resisting the urge to bend too far forwards in your spine. Exhale to rise back up with resistance. Don't rush. Repeat a total of 6 times.

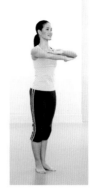

14 Return to Pilates stance, with your arms folded in front at chest height (see inset). Press down firmly into the floor with the balls o your feet so your heels rise up for 3 counts. Lower down with control. Continue for 6 repetitions, exhaling as you rise and inhaling as you lower.

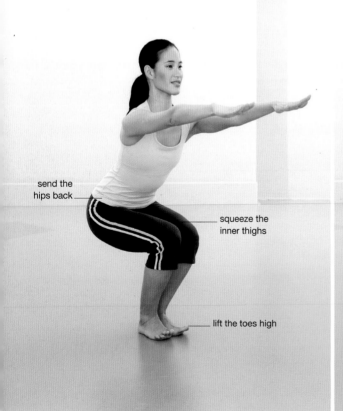

send the hips back

squeeze the inner thighs

lift the toes high

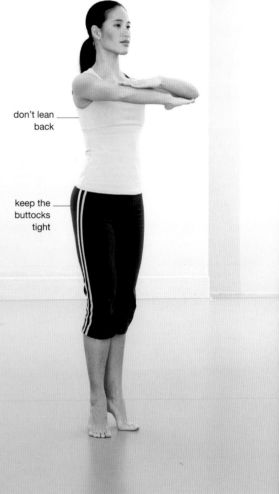

don't lean back

keep the buttocks tight

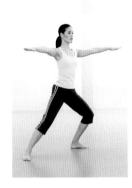

15 Once again, stand in Pilates stance, arms out to your sides. Lunge forwards with your left leg, transferring all your weight onto it (see inset). Keep your right leg firmly planted into the floor. Drag your left foot back to your right foot to start again. Inhale to lunge and exhale to pull back 4 times on each leg.

16 Return to Pilates stance, with your arms reaching out to the sides. Lunge sideways with your left leg (see inset), then drag the leg home, straightening it as quickly as possible to activate the upper inner thighs. Repeat 3 more times. Repeat with your other leg to the side.

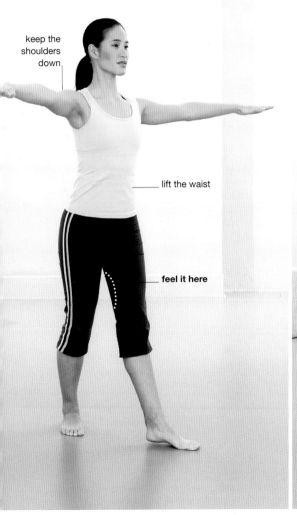

keep the shoulders down

lift the waist

feel it here

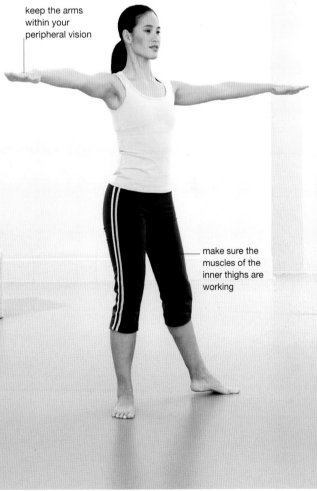

keep the arms within your peripheral vision

make sure the muscles of the inner thighs are working

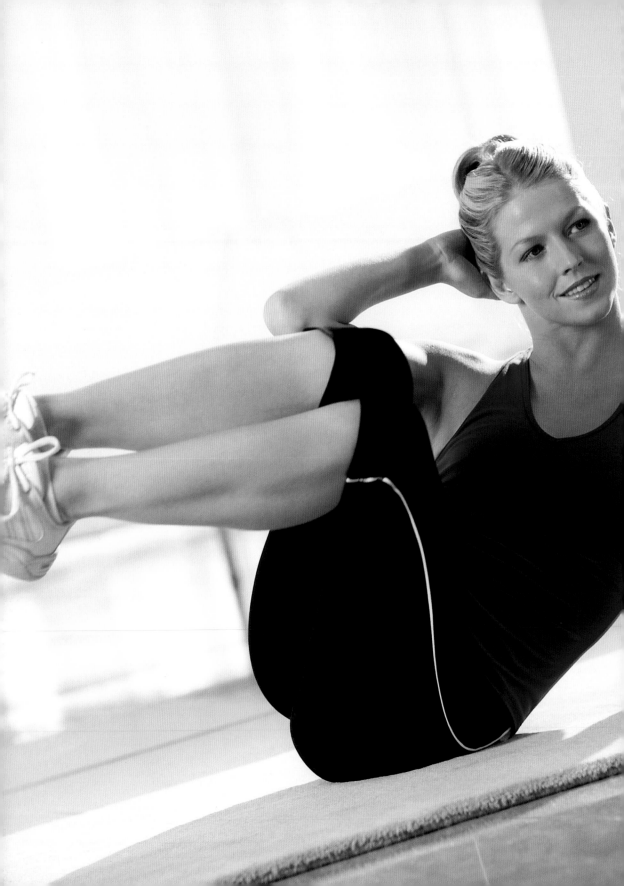

>> **15**minute

abs
workout

Joan Pagano

>> **focus** on the belly

View the paintings and sculptures in any art gallery or museum and what do you notice? Women have bellies – it's a fact of nature. There are many factors influencing the size and shape of your belly, but one thing is certain: a healthy lifestyle has a positive effect in every case.

Genetics determine your physical framework, including where you will carry body fat (apple or pear shape). All healthy people have fat reserves necessary for proper functioning of their bodies. Fat tends to accumulate in specific areas, and your personal genetics dictate where you will carry yours. Visceral fat found deep in the abdomen (apple) increases your risk of heart disease, but responds rapidly to diet and exercise.

Differences between the sexes can also play a role. Women typically have a higher percentage of body fat compared with men. This is designed to store the energy needed to nourish a foetus and then a baby. Structurally, a woman's pelvis is tilted a little more forwards than a man's so that during pregnancy there is less pressure on the organs since some of the baby's weight is carried by the abdominal muscles. This anterior tilt of the pelvis gives the impression that the lower belly is slightly pushed out, creating a "pot belly".

Age-related changes occur that affect the shape of our mid-section over time. "Middle-aged spread" and "spare tyres" typically occur after child-bearing as we approach the menopausal years. With advancing age, postural changes can cause spinal curves to become more exaggerated and push the belly forwards.

Many other factors may come into play. Weight gain and stress both influence the size of the belly; repeated pregnancies can affect muscle and skin tone; abdominal surgery can cause a loss of muscle strength, scar tissue, and an

> ## >> **exercise for** a smaller belly
>
> - **If your abs are toned** but have a layer of belly fat over them, add 30 minutes of cardio most days of the week to burn calories and reduce fat.
>
> - **If you do not have excess belly fat,** but lack of muscle tone causes your belly to hang, you should concentrate on the abs routines to firm up.
>
> - **If you are both** lacking muscle tone and carrying excess fat, step up both cardio (as above) and abs routines. Begin with the Crunch routine.

accumulation of fluids. Exercise can help improve many of these.

Before you begin, it is helpful to assess your individual issues and focus on the changes that you can make. Then establish a starting point for your programme (see Crunch Assessment pp64–65 and Safety Issues, pp4–5). Set realistic goals and measure your progress periodically.

So many factors influence the size and shape of your belly, including genetic predisposition, age, and lifestyle habits (physical activity and diet).

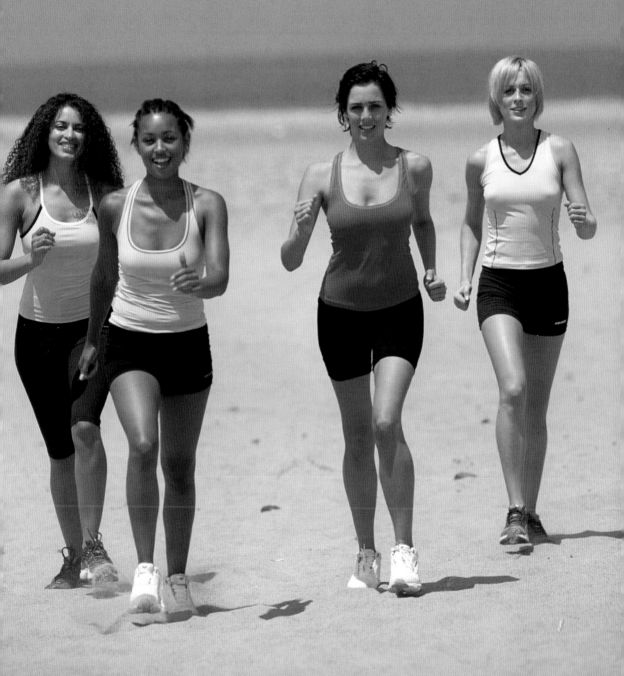

>> **the anatomy** of your abs

The core region of the body is very complex and technically consists of the collective muscles that control your trunk. The abdominals are central to the core region and work in concert with the erector spinae muscles of the spine to provide stability to the torso.

The abdominals consist of four muscle groups – the rectus abdominis, the internal and external obliques and the transversus abdominis. They are layered, overlapping, and connected to each other. They run vertically, diagonally and horizontally and often function synergistically.

The rectus abdominis is best known as the coveted "six-pack" muscle, which describes the

THE CORE MUSCLES

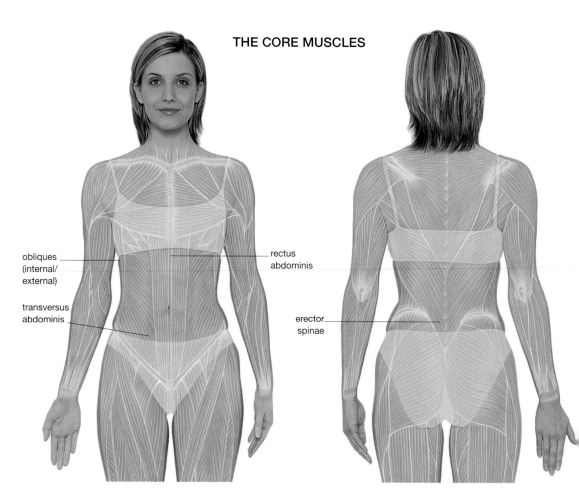

obliques (internal/external)

transversus abdominis

rectus abdominis

erector spinae

sections that develop when this muscle is toned. It is the most superficial muscle of the abdomen, running vertically from the sternum to the pubic bone. It functions to flex the spine and stabilize the pelvis as you walk.

The internal/external obliques are found on the sides of the core area and perform multiple functions. When they contract on one side of the body they rotate the trunk (as in the Side Crunch, see p73) and laterally flex the body (as in the Side Plank, see p111). When they contract on both sides of the body simultaneously, they assist in flexing the spine and compressing the abdomen (as in the Pelvic Tilt, see p71).

When it is toned, the transversus abdominis acts as a natural girdle, flattening the abdomen and supporting the low back. It runs horizontally around your mid-section and is the deepest abdominal muscle. This muscle works with the internal/external obliques to stabilize the pelvis in neutral position, as in the 90–90 exercise (see p104).

The erector spinae – the spinal extensors – run the length of the spine. Back extensions trigger this group (as in the Back Extension using the beach ball, see p95), strengthening the muscles for greater trunk support. In plank positions (see p151), the erector spinae function with the abdominals to stabilize the torso in the horizontal position.

Like any muscle group, the core muscles require 24 to 48 hours' recovery time between workouts. Although they are primarily endurance muscles, which recover quickly from an abundance of work, they still need time to rest, recover, and rebuild. The result will be added strength.

TARGETING CORE MUSCLES

Do your abs workouts 3 to 4 times a week on nonconsecutive days. Each routine gives you a balanced workout for the abs and spinal muscles. You can do multiple workouts on any given day, but must allow a day of rest before repeating them. The table below shows you which specific muscles are worked by each exercise.

CRUNCH	BEACH BALL	CORE BASICS
Rectus abdominis	**Rectus abdominis**	**Rectus abdominis**
Short Crunch, p71	Roll-back and Lift, p87	Roll-back, p107
Neutral Crunch, p72	Pullover Crunch, p89	**Transversus abdominis**
Long Crunch, p72	Reverse Crunch Combo, p90	Pelvic Tilt, p103
Diamond Crunch, p74		Straight-leg Lowering, p103
Reverse Crunch, p75	**Transversus abdominis**	90–90, p104
90–90 Crunch, p76	Reverse Crunch Combo, p90	Alternating Kicks, p104
Crunch and Dip, p76	Toe Tap, p92	Double-leg Lowering, p106
Bicycle, p77	Ball Transfer, pp92-93	**Obliques**
Transversus abdominis	**Obliques**	Knee Drop, p105
Pelvic Tilt, p71	Side Twist, p88	Spiral Ab Twist, p107
Crunch and Dip, p76	Side Reach, p89	Twisting Roll-back, p108
Obliques	Trunk Twist, p91	Side Plank, p111
Side Crunch, p73	Balancing Side Crunch, p93	**Erector spinae**
Torso Twist, p75	**Erector spinae**	Kneeling Lift, p109
Bicycle, p77	Forearm Plank, p94	Forearm Plank, p109
Erector spinae	Back Extension, p95	
Arm and Leg Lift, p77		
Press-up, p78		

>> **crunch** assessment

The crunch is the classic abs exercise, targeting the rectus abdominis muscle that runs from the sternum to the pubic bone. It is a versatile exercise, suitable for beginners or more advanced exercisers. It also ranks as one of the most effective for strengthening the abdomen.

The function of the rectus muscle is to flex the spine, and in the crunch you do not perform more than 30 degrees of spinal flexion (which refers to how high you lift your upper torso off the floor), even if you can raise your torso higher. This range of motion isolates the muscle, keeping the work in the rectus. If you lift higher, as in a full sit-up, for example, you activate other muscles, primarily the hip flexors in the front of the thigh. In addition to being a more effective isolation exercise than the full sit-up, the crunch places less stress on the low back and is therefore safer.

It is useful to have an objective measure of your starting level of abdominal fitness. Together with your health and medical information, a fitness assessment helps define your goals in an exercise programme. Establishing a baseline also enables you to measure your improvement. One way to measure muscular fitness is to count how many repetitions you can perform. Do the crunch test as described below. Write down your results, make a note of the date, and after two months of training, repeat the assessment.

To get the most from your workout, use proper form and execution of the crunch. Concentrate on perfecting the technique and apply it to each repetition. Mental focus also enhances the outcome – think about feeling the abdominal muscle tightening, strength coming from the core centre, lifting from the chest, head relaxed in your hands.

Preparation for the crunch

Make a cradle for your head by spreading your fingertips and supporting the base of your skull (see opposite, top right). Bend your fingers slightly and let the weight of your head rest in your hands. Keep your chin lifted, as if you were holding an orange under it (measure the distance with your fist, as in the photograph opposite, top left). Keep your elbows wide to reduce any tendency to pull on your neck.

With your low back relaxed in neutral alignment, engage the rectus abdominis by tightening the connection between the ribs and the hips. Keep tension in the muscle as you lift your chest to the ceiling, shoulder blades clearing the floor. Maintain the tension as you lower your shoulder blades to

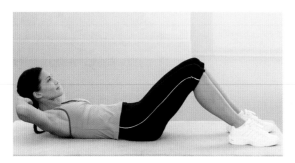

Neutral crunch
Count how many neutral crunches you can do consecutively without resting. Remember, this is not a full sit-up. Lift your shoulders no higher than 30 degrees off the mat.

Your score

Excellent	50 or more
Good	35–49 reps
Fair	20–34 reps
Poor	fewer than 20 reps

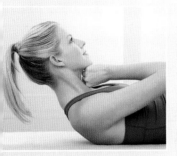

Fist under chin
Use your fist under your chin to gauge the correct alignment of the head. Always think, "Chin up".

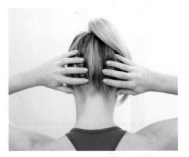

Position of hands on head Spread your fingers at the base of your skull to create a cradle for holding your head. Remember to relax your neck in your hands.

the floor and, without resting at the bottom, immediately repeat the lift. Keep drawing the ribs to the pelvis – think of "scooping" out the abdomen. Learn to breathe while you are drawing in, holding tension in the muscle – inhale first, then exhale as you lift up. Use slow, controlled movements and work the entire range of motion. It's quality not quantity that counts!

The weight of your head and upper torso provide resistance in the crunch. You can increase the intensity by

slowing the action, adding holds (as in the Long Crunch, see p72 and the Diamond Crunch, see p74), or by adding external resistance. In the Beach Ball workout (see pp84–97), for instance, a simple unweighted ball will do just fine; but you can increase the resistance for muscle strengthening by using a weighted ball of 1.4–1.8kg (3–4 pounds) – my favourite are filled with gel. Although there are heavier balls available, it is better to use one of this weight and maintain proper form, being careful not to use momentum in the movements.

Connecting ribs to hips Set your abs before you move. Think of connecting the ribs to the hips. Maintain this connection, drawing ribs to pelvis, while you perform crunches.

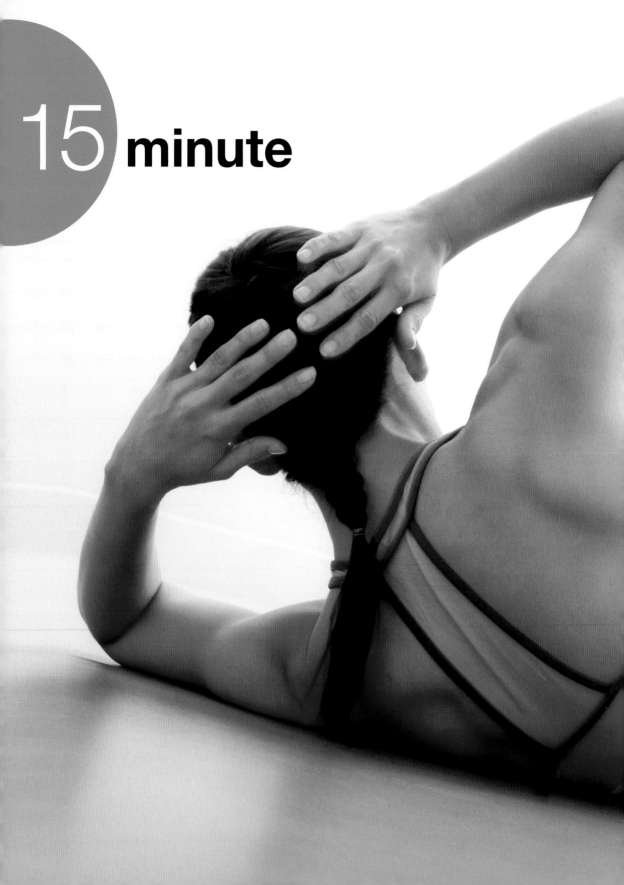

15 minute

crunch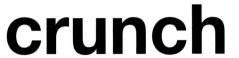

Shape up with the one of the
most effective ab exercises
Perfect the classic crunch

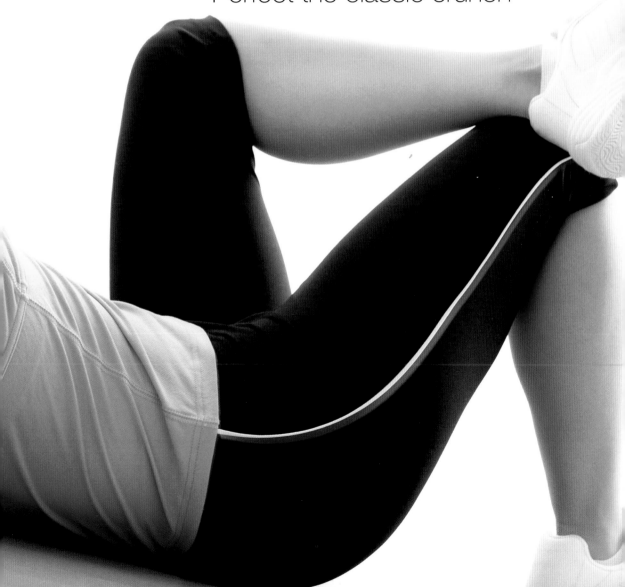

>> march in place/step-touch in

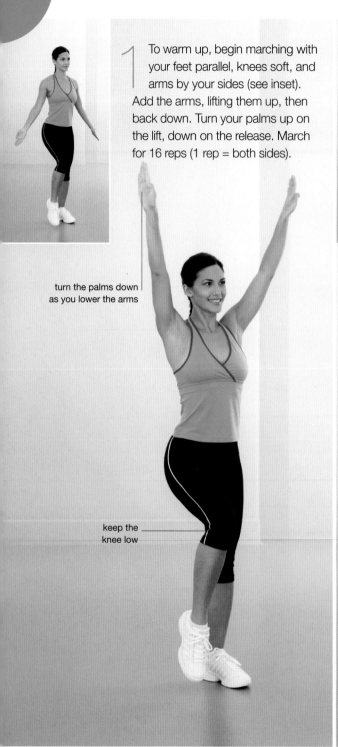

1 To warm up, begin marching with your feet parallel, knees soft, and arms by your sides (see inset). Add the arms, lifting them up, then back down. Turn your palms up on the lift, down on the release. March for 16 reps (1 rep = both sides).

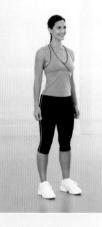

2 Step one leg to the side, arms by your sides (see inset). Step the other leg in, touching your feet together, bending your elbows to that side and swinging your hands to shoulder height. Repeat, moving from side to side, for 8 reps.

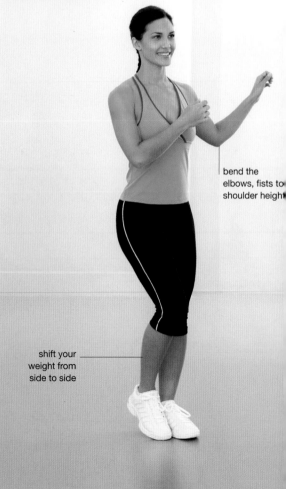

turn the palms down as you lower the arms

keep the knee low

bend the elbows, fists to shoulder height

shift your weight from side to side

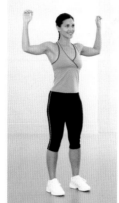

3 Step your feet apart, arms by your sides (see inset). Swing both arms to one side at shoulder height, coming up on the toes of the opposite foot. Circle your arms down to the other side and reach out with the tapping leg. Repeat, alternating sides for 8 reps.

4 With legs apart, raise your arms sideways to shoulder height. Bend your elbows to 90 degrees, palms forwards (see inset). Keeping your back straight, bend one knee to hip height. Rotate your torso, bringing the opposite elbow towards the raised knee. Repeat, alternating sides for 8 reps.

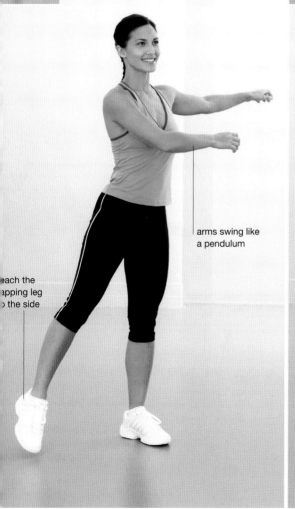

arms swing like a pendulum

each the apping leg the side

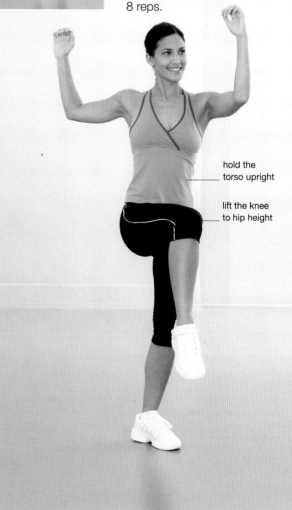

hold the torso upright

lift the knee to hip height

>> hamstring curl/body sway

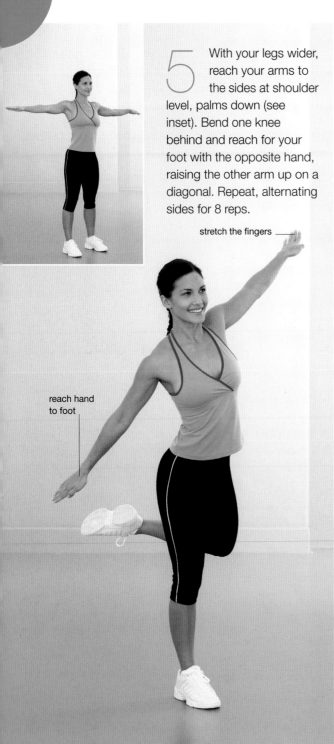

5 With your legs wider, reach your arms to the sides at shoulder level, palms down (see inset). Bend one knee behind and reach for your foot with the opposite hand, raising the other arm up on a diagonal. Repeat, alternating sides for 8 reps.

stretch the fingers

reach hand to foot

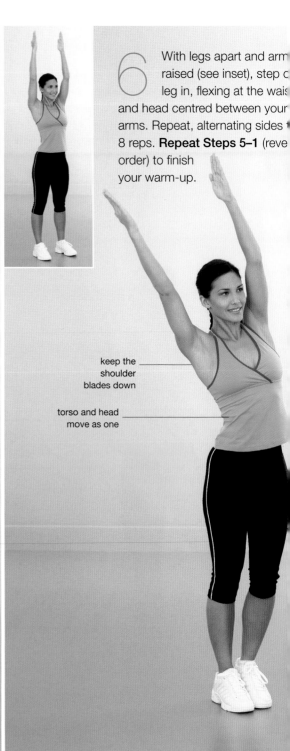

6 With legs apart and arm raised (see inset), step c leg in, flexing at the wais and head centred between your arms. Repeat, alternating sides 8 reps. **Repeat Steps 5–1** (reve order) to finish your warm-up.

keep the shoulder blades down

torso and head move as one

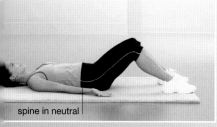

spine in neutral

7 Lie on your back in neutral position with knees bent at 90 degrees, feet flat on the floor and arms by your sides, palms up. Inhale, fill your belly with air (see inset). Then exhale forcefully, pulling your abs in tight and, with one fluid motion, flatten your low back to the floor. Hold for a moment, then release and repeat 10 times.

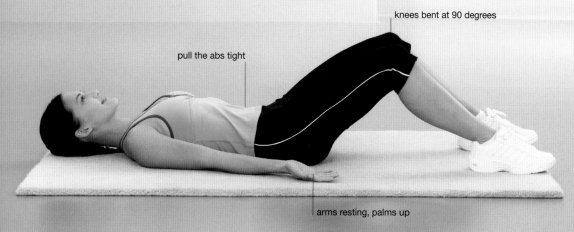

knees bent at 90 degrees

pull the abs tight

arms resting, palms up

8 From neutral position, move your feet in close to your buttocks, connect the ribs to the hips, then place your hands behind your head (see inset). Inhale first, then exhale, scooping out your abdomen, belly button to spine, as you lift your shoulder blades 30 degrees off the floor. Release, slowly lowering your shoulders (but not your head) to the floor. Repeat 10 times.

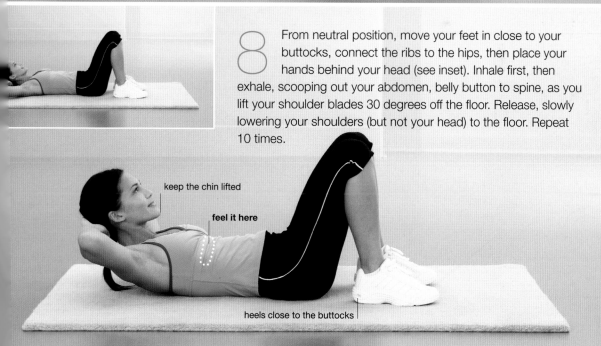

keep the chin lifted

feel it here

heels close to the buttocks

>> neutral crunch/long crunch

9 Move your feet forwards to neutral position. Tighten your abdomen by drawing your ribs towards your pelvis. Pick up the pace and continue to lift and lower your shoulders rhythmically, exhaling as you lift and inhaling as you release, maintaining tension in your abs throughout the movement. Repeat 10 times.

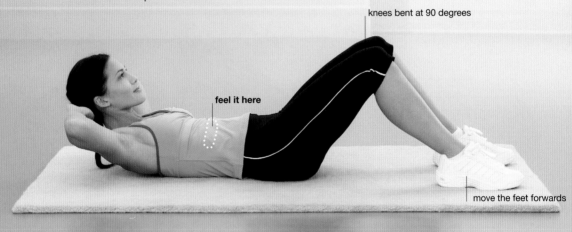

knees bent at 90 degrees

feel it here

move the feet forwards

10 Extend your legs, keeping a slight bend in your knees. Inhale first, then exhale and pull *in* when you crunch *up*. Add a hold at the top of the movement and release slowly. Learn to keep tension in the muscle while you continue to breathe. Repeat 10 times, then stretch out, arms and legs long.

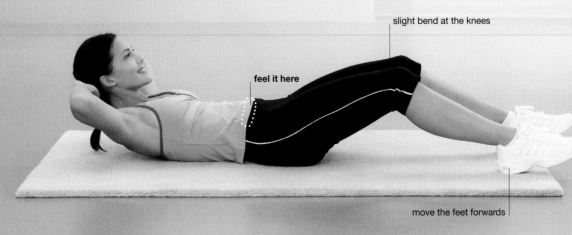

slight bend at the knees

feel it here

move the feet forwards

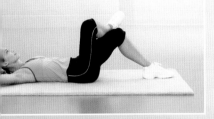

11 From neutral position, cross one ankle over the opposite knee, hands behind your head (see inset). With elbows wide, inhale, then exhale and twist one shoulder towards the opposite knee. Pause, then slowly release without resting your head on the floor. Repeat 5 times on each side.

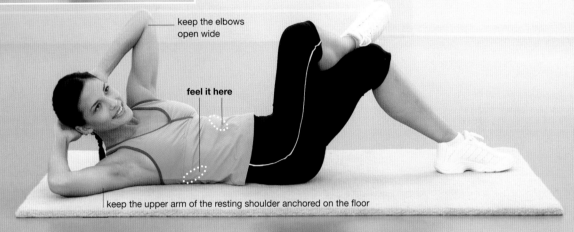

keep the elbows open wide

feel it here

keep the upper arm of the resting shoulder anchored on the floor

12 Reach out long, extending your arms and legs. Take a deep breath in and stretch out as far as you can. Cross one ankle over the other and take the wrist on the same side in your other hand. Pull to the opposite side, stretching out the entire side of your torso. Pause, then change sides and repeat.

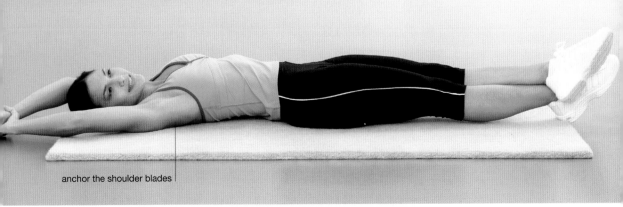

anchor the shoulder blades

>> **bridge/diamond crunch**

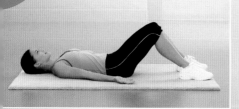

13 Return to neutral position and begin with a Pelvic Tilt (see inset). Then inhale, exhale and, starting at the base of your spine, peel your back off the floor, one vertebra at a time, until your torso forms a straight line from knees to shoulders. Inhale as you release down, rolling through the curve in your low back. Repeat 5 times.

torso aligned from the shoulders to the knees

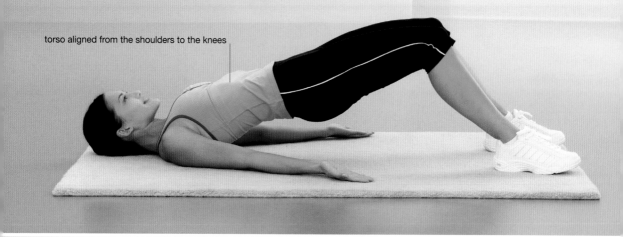

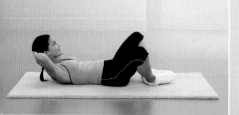

14 Lie with your knees out to the sides, soles of your feet together, as close to your body as possible. Connect your ribs to your hips, then rest your head in your hands and tighten your abs. Exhale as you lift your shoulder blades (see inset). Extend your arms towards your feet, crunching up higher. Return hands behind your head, release down and repeat 6 times.

crunch higher as you reach

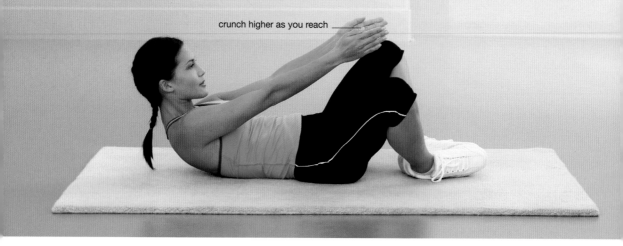

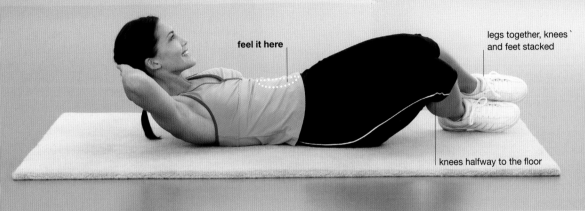

15 Return to neutral position, hands behind head, and bring your legs together, knees and feet touching. Reset your abs. Slowly rotate your pelvis to one side, moving your knees halfway to the floor (see inset). Inhale, then exhale and crunch up towards the ceiling 10 times. Relax your knees to the floor and rest in a Spinal Twist (see p88), turning the head in the opposite direction, then repeat to the other side.

feel it here

legs together, knees and feet stacked

knees halfway to the floor

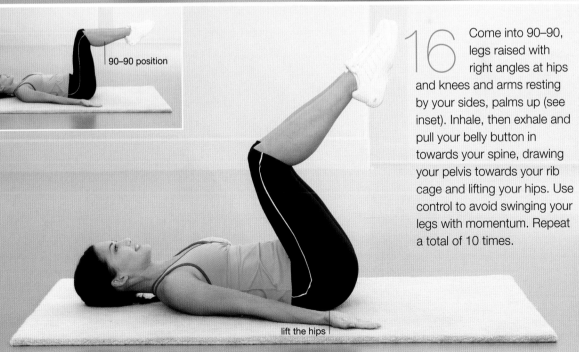

90–90 position

16 Come into 90–90, legs raised with right angles at hips and knees and arms resting by your sides, palms up (see inset). Inhale, then exhale and pull your belly button in towards your spine, drawing your pelvis towards your rib cage and lifting your hips. Use control to avoid swinging your legs with momentum. Repeat a total of 10 times.

lift the hips

>> 90–90 crunch/crunch and dip

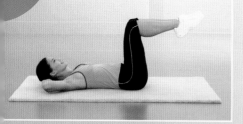

17 Still in 90–90, place your hands behind your head and tighten the connection between your ribs and your hips (see inset). Exhale as you lift your shoulder blades, eyes on the ceiling, chin lifted. Repeat 10 times. When you have finished, hug your knees into your chest and rest.

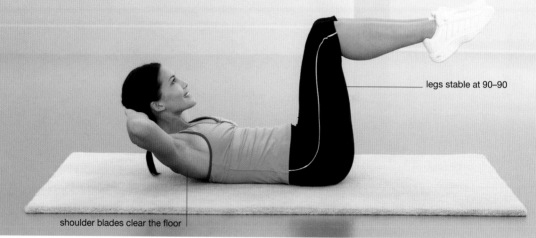

legs stable at 90–90

shoulder blades clear the floor

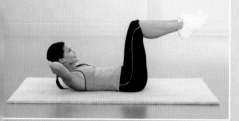

18 Resume 90–90 with your hands behind your head, exhale and do an upper torso crunch (see inset). Hold it while you inhale and dip your toes to the mat. Exhale and return legs to 90–90, then inhale and release the crunch. Repeat 10 times, then hug your knees into your chest for a breather.

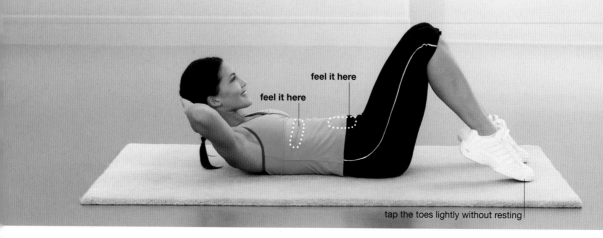

feel it here

feel it here

tap the toes lightly without resting

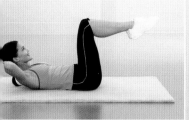

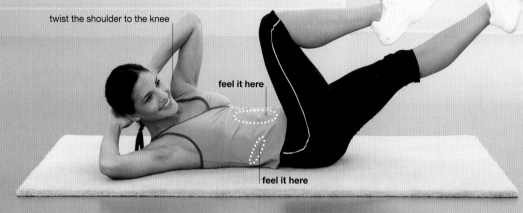

19 Return to 90–90, hands behind your head. Start with an upper torso crunch (see inset), then exhale as you twist one elbow to the opposite knee, bringing your knee into your chest and extending your other leg towards the floor. Inhale back to centre and go to the other side. Alternate sides for 5 reps, keeping your shoulder blades lifted. Reach out long to stretch.

twist the shoulder to the knee

feel it here

feel it here

20 Lying face down, extend your arms, palms down. Scoop out your abdomen and press your pubic bone into the floor (see inset). With your forehead still resting, exhale and lift one arm and the opposite leg, lengthening the limbs as you lift up. Repeat for 5 reps.

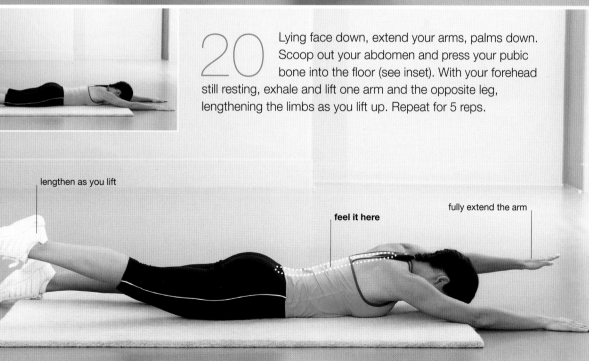

lengthen as you lift

feel it here

fully extend the arm

>> **press-up/sphinx**

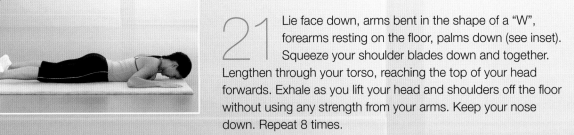

21 Lie face down, arms bent in the shape of a "W", forearms resting on the floor, palms down (see inset). Squeeze your shoulder blades down and together. Lengthen through your torso, reaching the top of your head forwards. Exhale as you lift your head and shoulders off the floor without using any strength from your arms. Keep your nose down. Repeat 8 times.

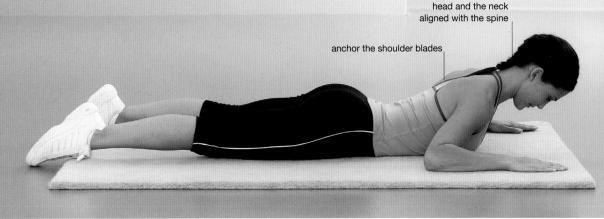

head and the neck aligned with the spine

anchor the shoulder blades

22 Lying face down, elbows bent with forearms resting on the mat, anchor your shoulder blades as you lift your chest, sliding your elbows forwards to be directly under your shoulders. Pull your ribs away from your hips, stretching your abdomen (see inset). With your shoulders square to the front, turn your head to one side and hold; then to the other.

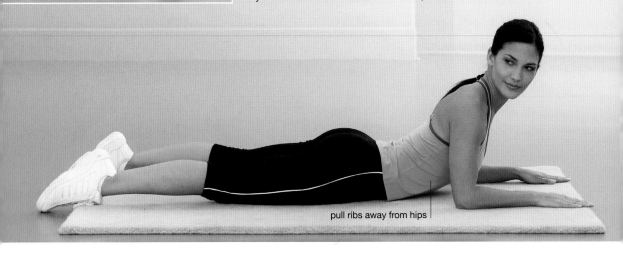

pull ribs away from hips

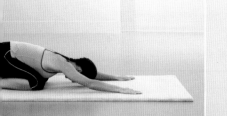

23 Sit back on your heels and bend forwards, forehead reaching to mat, arms stretching centre (see inset). Walk your hands to one side, keeping your head centred between your elbows, then to the other side. Use your breath to deepen the stretch: let your body sink into the position with every exhale.

head centred between the elbows

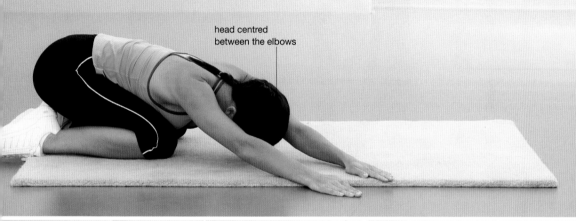

24 Kneel on all fours, wrists under shoulders, knees under hips (see inset). From neutral, lift your head and hips up, curving your spine into a "C".

lift the hips up

lift the head up

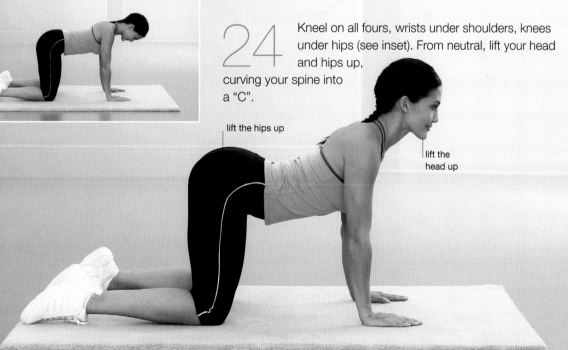

>> spinal arch/ear tilt

25 Now arch your spine, rounding your back up to the ceiling by tucking your hips under and dropping your head between your arms. Repeat each curve and arch 4 times, breathing naturally throughout.

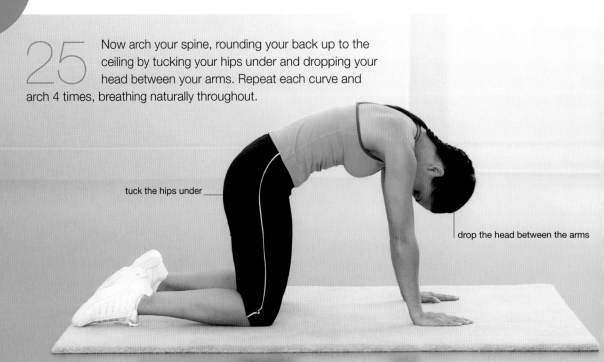

tuck the hips under

drop the head between the arms

26 Sit up tall, hips firmly planted on the floor, legs crossed comfortably in front. Anchor your shoulder blades. Tilt your ear to your shoulder, using your hand on the side of your head to gently deepen the stretch, while you reach down with your other hand to create a dynamic opposition. Hold and breathe.

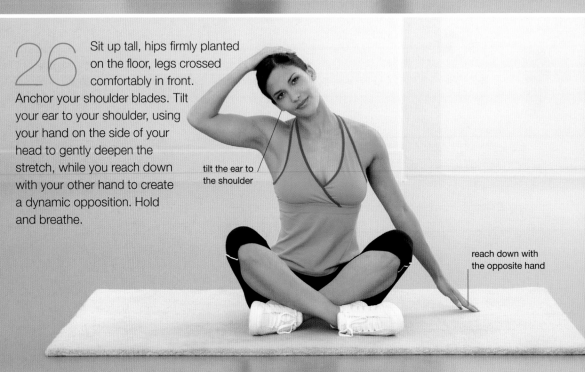

tilt the ear to the shoulder

reach down with the opposite hand

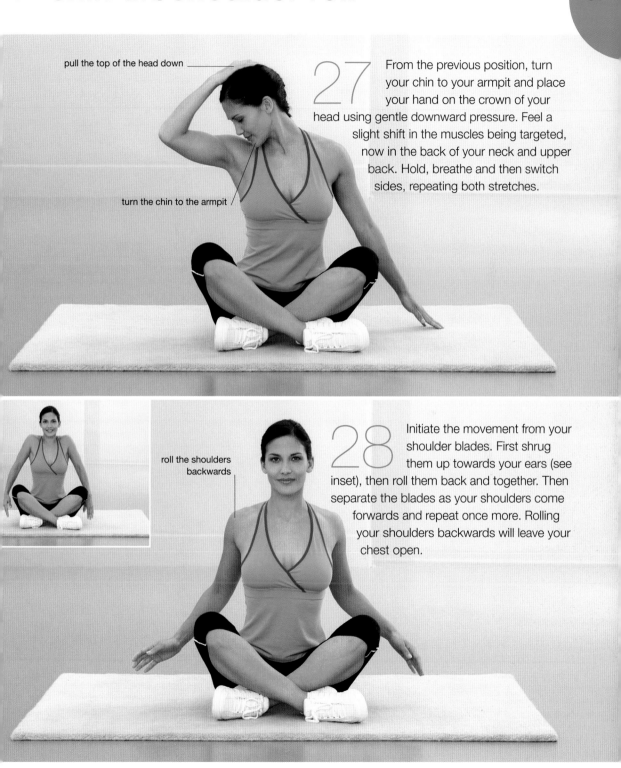

pull the top of the head down

turn the chin to the armpit

27 From the previous position, turn your chin to your armpit and place your hand on the crown of your head using gentle downward pressure. Feel a slight shift in the muscles being targeted, now in the back of your neck and upper back. Hold, breathe and then switch sides, repeating both stretches.

roll the shoulders backwards

28 Initiate the movement from your shoulder blades. First shrug them up towards your ears (see inset), then roll them back and together. Then separate the blades as your shoulders come forwards and repeat once more. Rolling your shoulders backwards will leave your chest open.

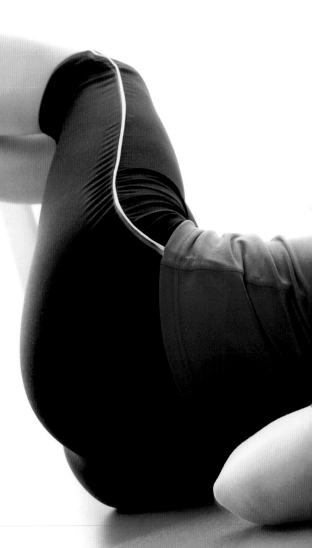

15 minute

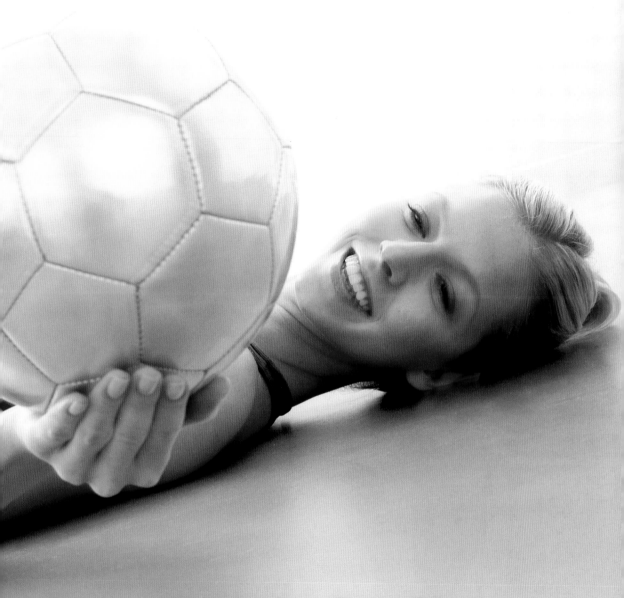

beach ball >>

Use a ball to add fun and resistance
Give new energy to traditional exercises

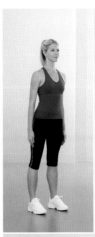

1 To warm up, begin marching with your feet parallel, knees soft, and arms by your sides (see inset). Add the arms, lifting them up, with palms up, then back down, with palms down. March for 16 reps (1 rep = both sides).

2 Step one leg to the side, arms by your sides. Step the other leg in, touching your feet together, bending your elbows to that side and swinging your hands to shoulder height. Repeat, moving from side to side, for 8 reps.

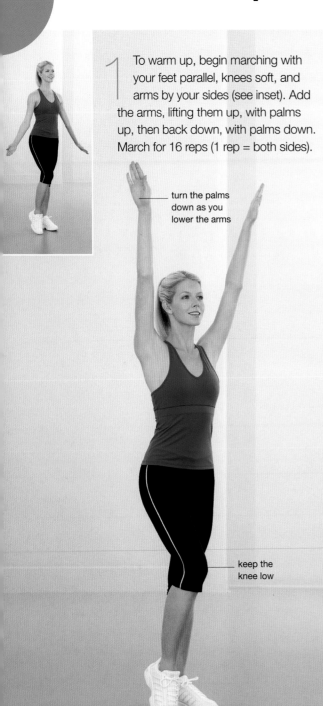

turn the palms down as you lower the arms

keep the knee low

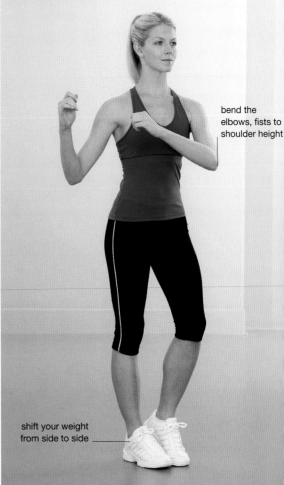

bend the elbows, fists to shoulder height

shift your weight from side to side

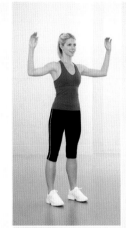

3 Step your feet apart, arms by your sides. Swing both arms to one side at shoulder height, coming up on the toes of the opposite foot. Circle your arms down to the other side and reach out with the tapping leg. Repeat, alternating sides for 8 reps.

4 With legs apart, raise the arms sideways, to shoulder height. Bend your elbows to 90 degrees, palms forwards. With a straight back, bend one knee to hip height. Rotate your torso, bringing the opposite elbow towards the raised knee. Repeat, alternating sides for 8 reps.

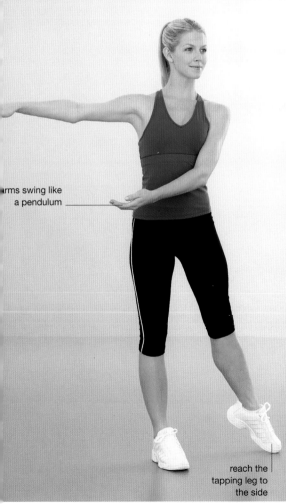

arms swing like a pendulum

reach the tapping leg to the side

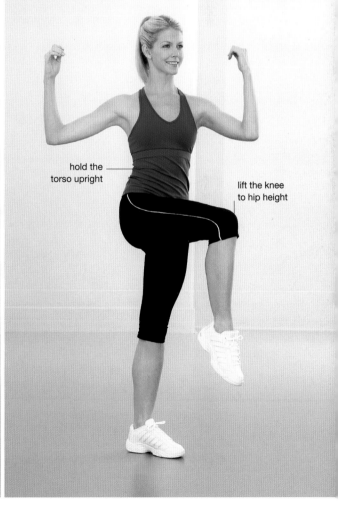

hold the torso upright

lift the knee to hip height

>> hamstring curl/body sway

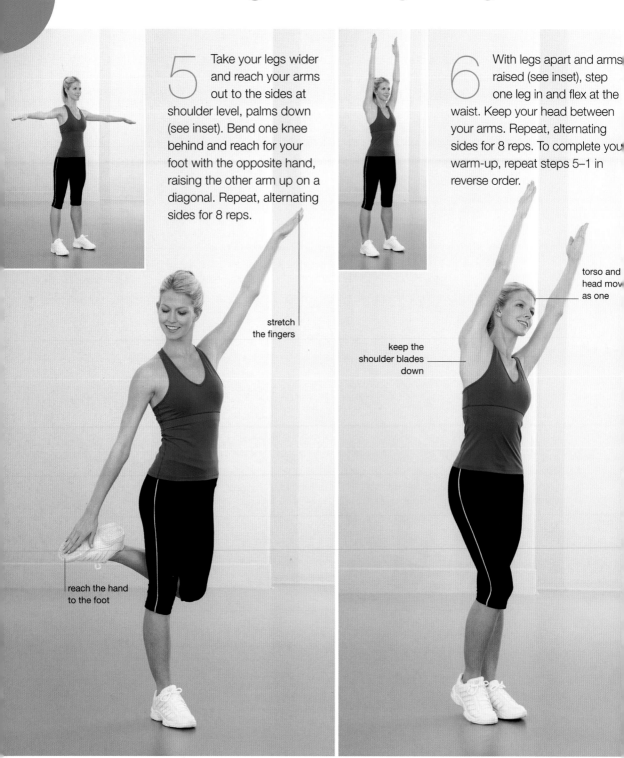

5 Take your legs wider and reach your arms out to the sides at shoulder level, palms down (see inset). Bend one knee behind and reach for your foot with the opposite hand, raising the other arm up on a diagonal. Repeat, alternating sides for 8 reps.

6 With legs apart and arms raised (see inset), step one leg in and flex at the waist. Keep your head between your arms. Repeat, alternating sides for 8 reps. To complete your warm-up, repeat steps 5–1 in reverse order.

stretch the fingers

reach the hand to the foot

keep the shoulder blades down

torso and head move as one

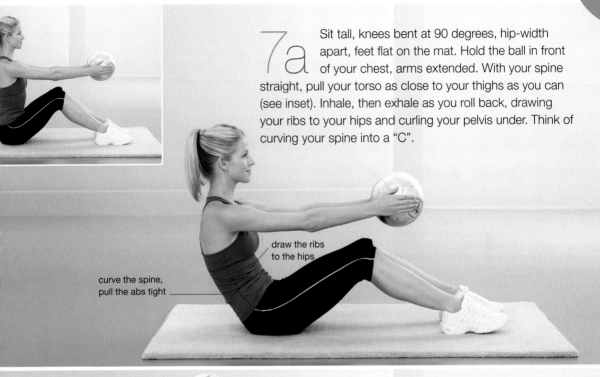

7a Sit tall, knees bent at 90 degrees, hip-width apart, feet flat on the mat. Hold the ball in front of your chest, arms extended. With your spine straight, pull your torso as close to your thighs as you can (see inset). Inhale, then exhale as you roll back, drawing your ribs to your hips and curling your pelvis under. Think of curving your spine into a "C".

draw the ribs
to the hips

curve the spine,
pull the abs tight

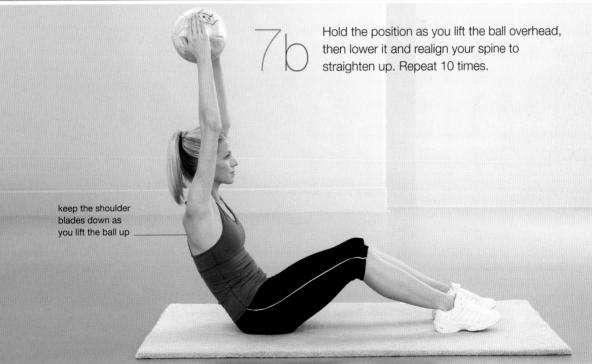

7b Hold the position as you lift the ball overhead, then lower it and realign your spine to straighten up. Repeat 10 times.

keep the shoulder
blades down as
you lift the ball up

>> side twist/spinal twist

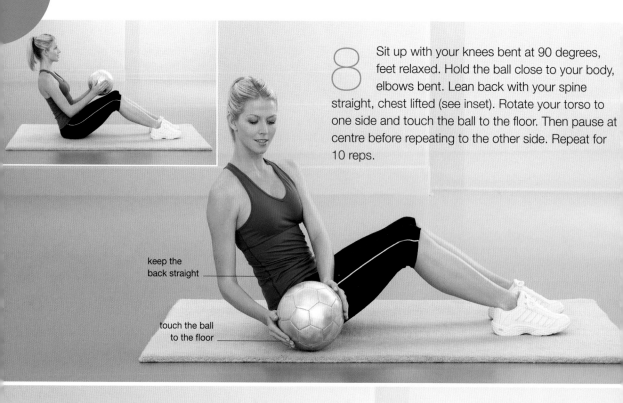

8 Sit up with your knees bent at 90 degrees, feet relaxed. Hold the ball close to your body, elbows bent. Lean back with your spine straight, chest lifted (see inset). Rotate your torso to one side and touch the ball to the floor. Then pause at centre before repeating to the other side. Repeat for 10 reps.

keep the back straight

touch the ball to the floor

9 Roll down to the floor, keeping your knees bent and set the ball aside. Stretch your arms out at shoulder level, with your palms facing up and rotate your knees to one side in a spinal twist. Turn your head the opposite way. Hold for a moment, then change sides.

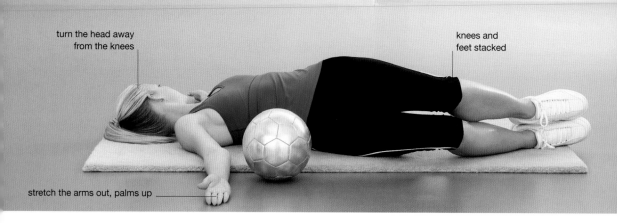

turn the head away from the knees

knees and feet stacked

stretch the arms out, palms up

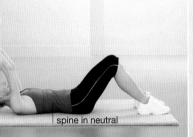

spine in neutral

10 Lie on your back in neutral position, knees bent at 90 degrees and feet flat on the floor. Hold the ball diagonally overhead with your shoulder blades anchored (see inset). Inhale, then exhale, keep your abs tight and lift your torso, reaching the ball to your knees. Release back without resting and repeat 10 times. Then rest and rock your head from side to side.

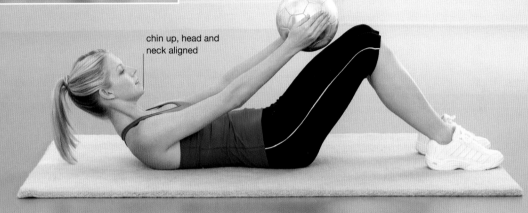

chin up, head and neck aligned

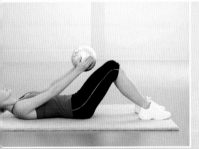

11 Lie on your back in the neutral position. Hold the ball towards your knees, arms straight (see inset). Inhale, then exhale and lift your shoulder blades, reaching the ball to one side. Hold. Pass through centre to the other side. Repeat for 8 reps, alternating sides. Finally, extend your legs and reach your arms long, with the ball behind your head. Rock your head from side to side to ease any tension in the neck.

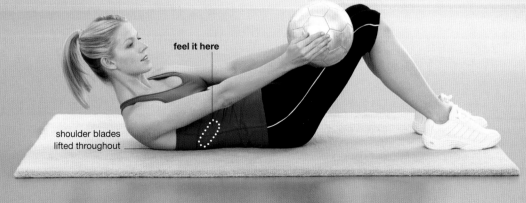

feel it here

shoulder blades lifted throughout

>> reverse crunch combo

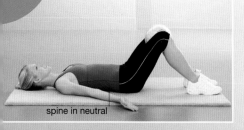

spine in neutral

12a

Place the ball between your knees and come into neutral position, arms by your sides, palms up (see inset). To initiate the Bridge, perform a Pelvic Tilt (see p71).

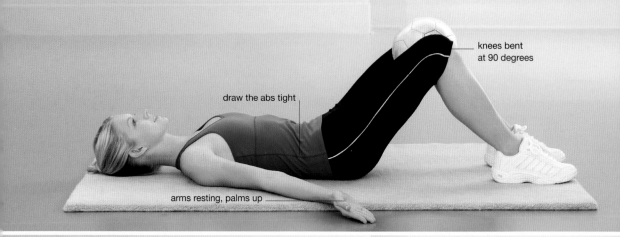

knees bent at 90 degrees

draw the abs tight

arms resting, palms up

12b

Complete the Bridge by lifting your hips until they form a straight line connecting your knees to your shoulders. Release, rolling down sequentially through your spine.

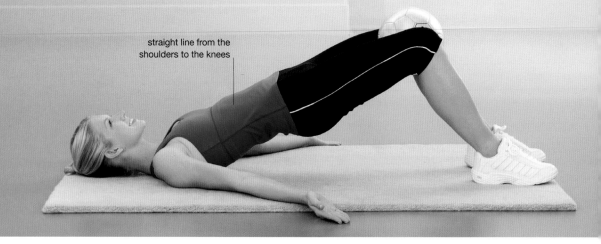

straight line from the shoulders to the knees

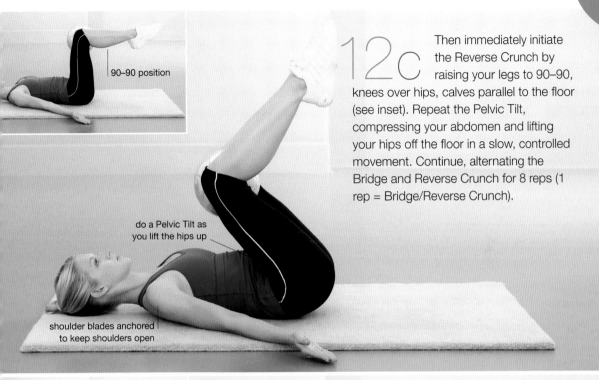

90–90 position

12c Then immediately initiate the Reverse Crunch by raising your legs to 90–90, knees over hips, calves parallel to the floor (see inset). Repeat the Pelvic Tilt, compressing your abdomen and lifting your hips off the floor in a slow, controlled movement. Continue, alternating the Bridge and Reverse Crunch for 8 reps (1 rep = Bridge/Reverse Crunch).

do a Pelvic Tilt as you lift the hips up

shoulder blades anchored to keep shoulders open

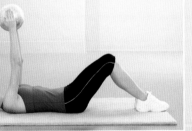

13 From neutral position, bring your legs together, knees and ankles touching. Hold the ball to the ceiling over your chest (see inset). Lower your knees to one side while you reach the ball to the other. Keep your knees and feet stacked as you rotate your pelvis. Repeat for 8 reps, alternating sides. Now set the ball down and do a Spinal Twist (see p88) to each side.

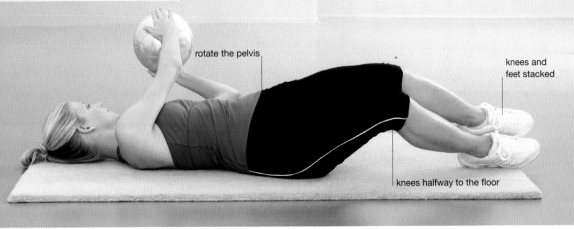

rotate the pelvis

knees and feet stacked

knees halfway to the floor

>> toe tap/ball transfer

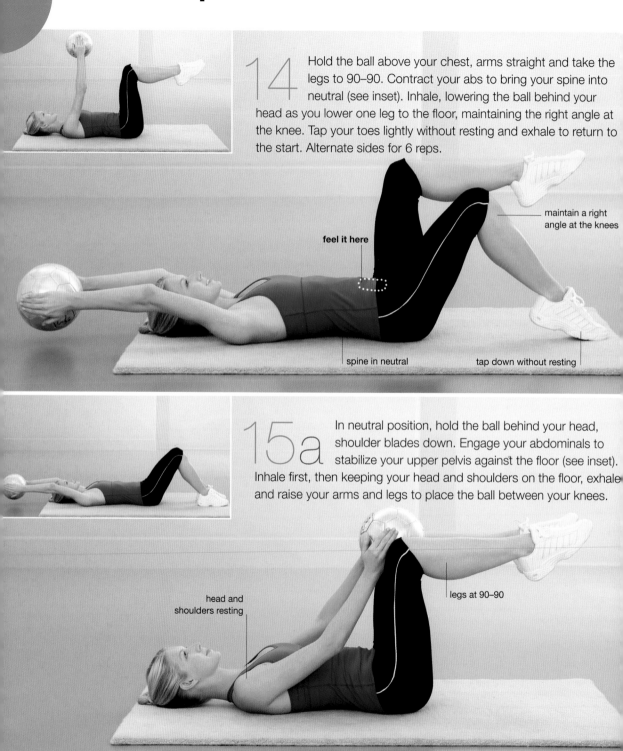

14 Hold the ball above your chest, arms straight and take the legs to 90–90. Contract your abs to bring your spine into neutral (see inset). Inhale, lowering the ball behind your head as you lower one leg to the floor, maintaining the right angle at the knee. Tap your toes lightly without resting and exhale to return to the start. Alternate sides for 6 reps.

maintain a right angle at the knees

feel it here

spine in neutral

tap down without resting

15a In neutral position, hold the ball behind your head, shoulder blades down. Engage your abdominals to stabilize your upper pelvis against the floor (see inset). Inhale first, then keeping your head and shoulders on the floor, exhale and raise your arms and legs to place the ball between your knees.

legs at 90–90

head and shoulders resting

15b Inhale, lowering your arms and feet towards the floor without arching your back. Tap toes down, then exhale as you lift your limbs again to grasp the ball in your hands and return to start. This is 1 rep. Repeat Steps 15a and 15b for a total of 5 reps, then stretch out long, holding the ball behind your head.

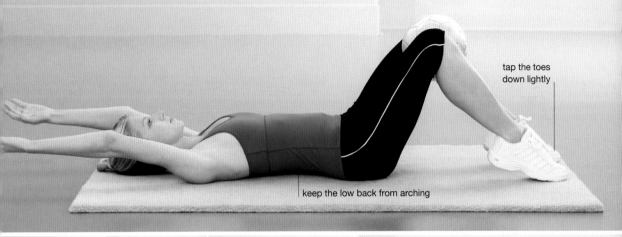

tap the toes down lightly

keep the low back from arching

16 In neutral position, place the ball under one foot and extend the other leg (see inset). With the hands behind the head and the elbows wide, exhale and lift the shoulder blade, twisting that shoulder towards the knee as the working leg bends to meet the elbow. Do this 10 times. Change sides and repeat.

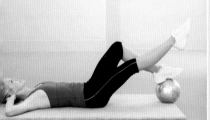

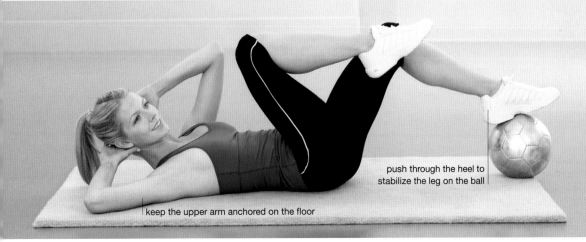

push through the heel to stabilize the leg on the ball

keep the upper arm anchored on the floor

17 Turn onto your stomach and draw your shoulder blades down and together. Lift your chest, position your elbows directly under your shoulders and hold the ball between your hands. Reach the top of your head to the ceiling while you breathe into the stretch, lengthening through the torso.

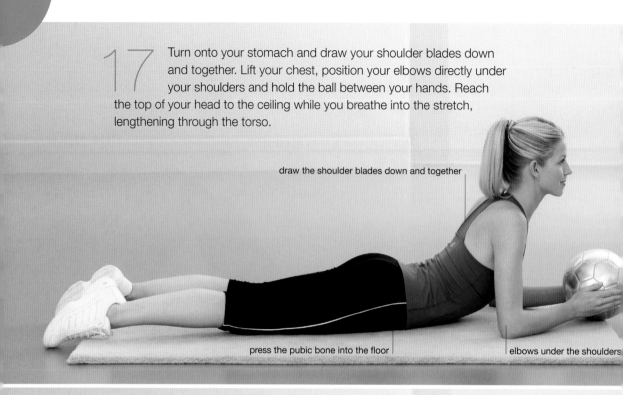

draw the shoulder blades down and together

press the pubic bone into the floor

elbows under the shoulders

18 From the Sphinx, with your shoulders anchored and still holding the ball, scoop out your abs and lift your hips, making a straight line from shoulder to knee. Keep your shoulder blades wide and apart, head and neck aligned with your spine. To increase the intensity, tuck your toes under and lift your knees.

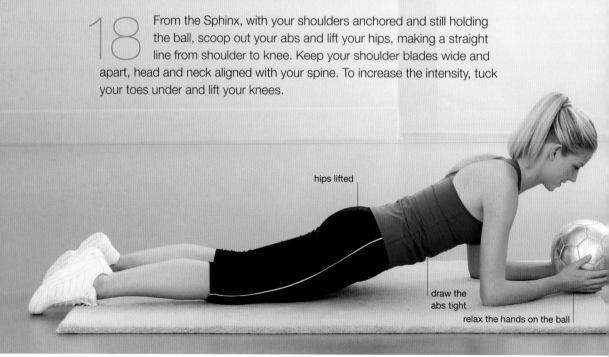

hips lifted

draw the abs tight

relax the hands on the ball

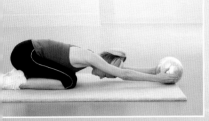

19 Bend your knees and reach back with your hips, curving your spine until your buttocks rest on your heels. At the same time, straighten your arms to the front, reaching the ball forwards and lower your forehead towards the floor (see inset). Then roll the ball to one side and, still reaching with it, hold the stretch. Repeat to the other side.

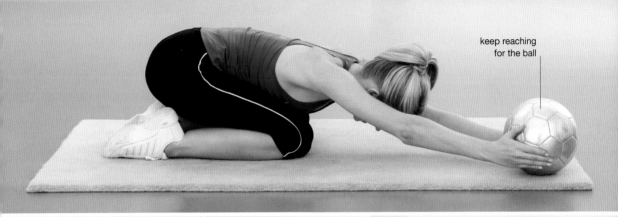

keep reaching for the ball

20 Holding the ball with both hands, slide forwards onto your stomach, legs hip-width apart. Move the ball to your low back, holding it with fingers pointing back, elbows bent to the ceiling (inset). Rest your forehead on the mat. Inhale, then exhale, lift your chest and straighten your arms, pressing the ball down your back. Inhale, then bend your arms to return. Repeat 10 times.

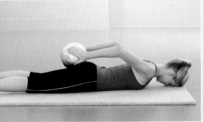

straighten the arms, reach the ball to the feet

feel it here

head and neck aligned with the spine

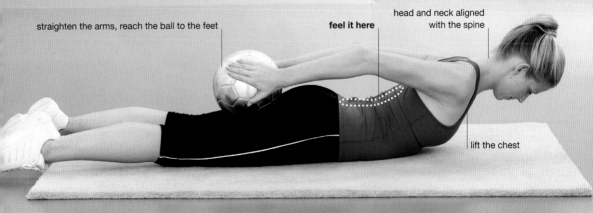

lift the chest

>> bridge stretch/low-back stretch

21 Turn onto your back, knees bent, feet on the floor. Lift your hips and place the ball under the sacrum, allowing it to support your body weight. Inhale and on the exhale feel the low back relax. Hold the ball with your hands if necessary. Take several deep breaths.

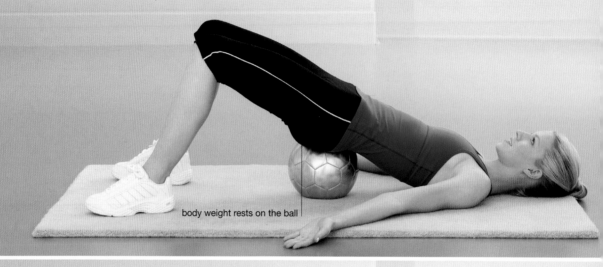

body weight rests on the ball

22 From the Bridge Stretch, bring one knee up over your chest and then the other. Separate the knees, still allowing the ball to support you. Continue to hold onto the ball or turn your palms up and rest your arms by your sides. With every exhale, let your body weight sink into the ball. To come out of the stretch, hold onto the ball and lower one leg at a time.

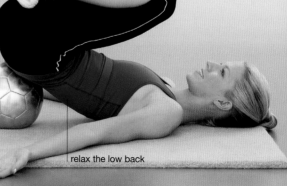

relax the low back

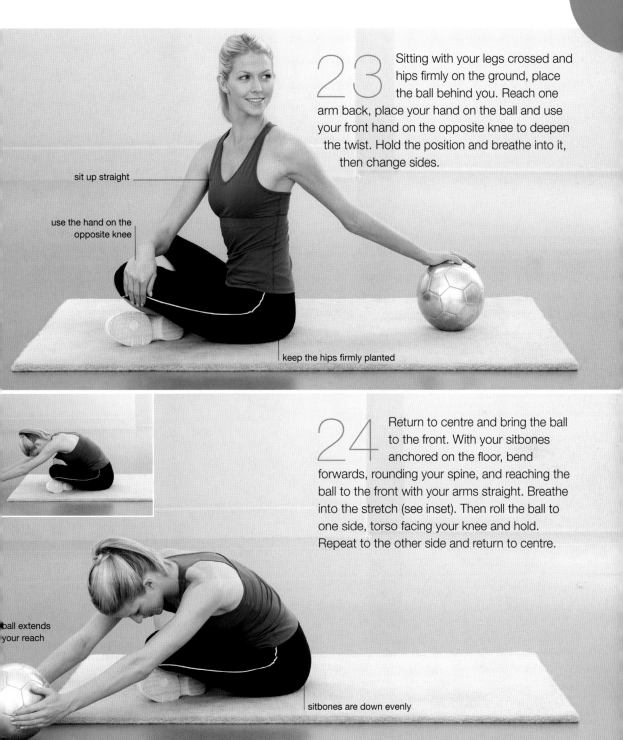

23 Sitting with your legs crossed and hips firmly on the ground, place the ball behind you. Reach one arm back, place your hand on the ball and use your front hand on the opposite knee to deepen the twist. Hold the position and breathe into it, then change sides.

sit up straight

use the hand on the opposite knee

keep the hips firmly planted

24 Return to centre and bring the ball to the front. With your sitbones anchored on the floor, bend forwards, rounding your spine, and reaching the ball to the front with your arms straight. Breathe into the stretch (see inset). Then roll the ball to one side, torso facing your knee and hold. Repeat to the other side and return to centre.

ball extends your reach

sitbones are down evenly

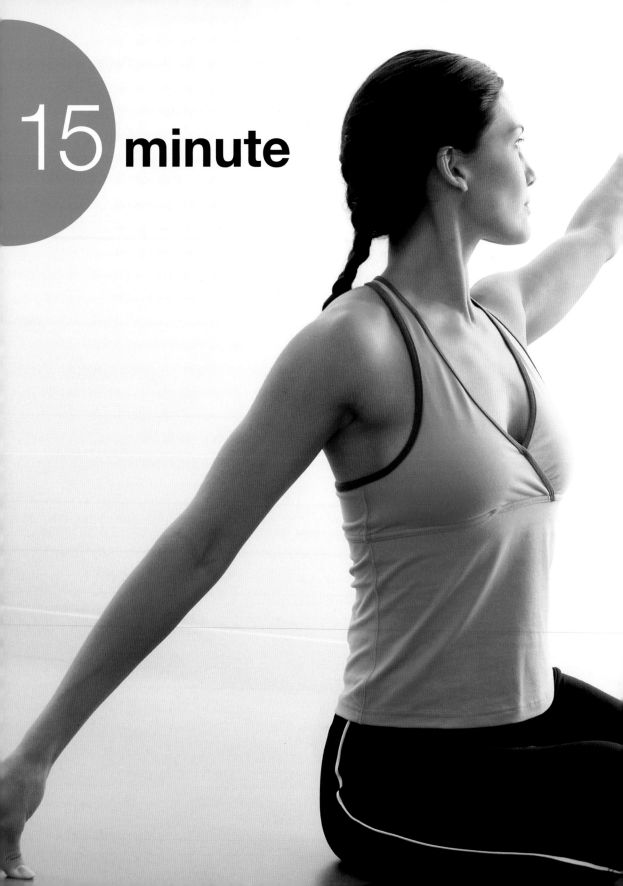

15 minute

Get in touch with your
deep abdominals
Flatten your belly

core basics >>

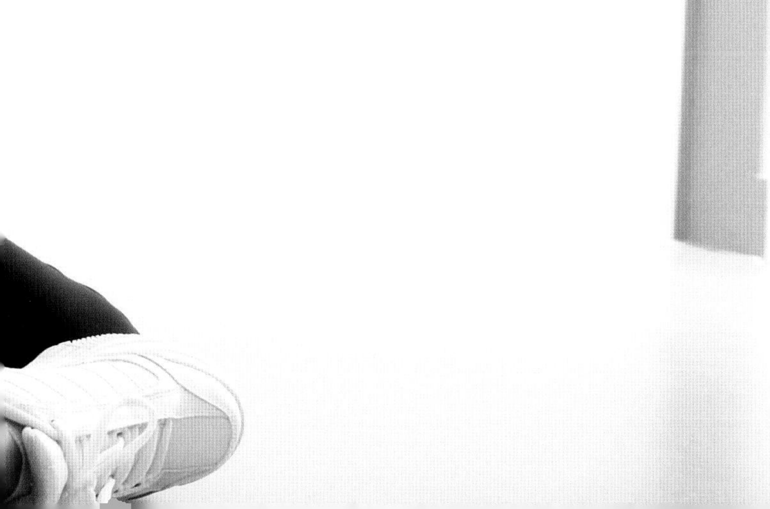

>> march in place/step-touch in

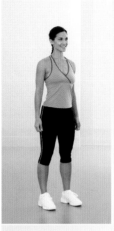

1 To warm up, begin marching with your feet parallel, knees soft, and arms by your sides (see inset). Add the arms, lifting them up, then back down. Turn your palms up on the lift, down on the release. March for 16 reps (1 rep = both sides).

2 Step one leg to the side, arms by your sides. Step the other leg in, touching your feet together, bending your elbows to that side and swinging your hands to shoulder height. Repeat, moving from side to side, for 8 reps.

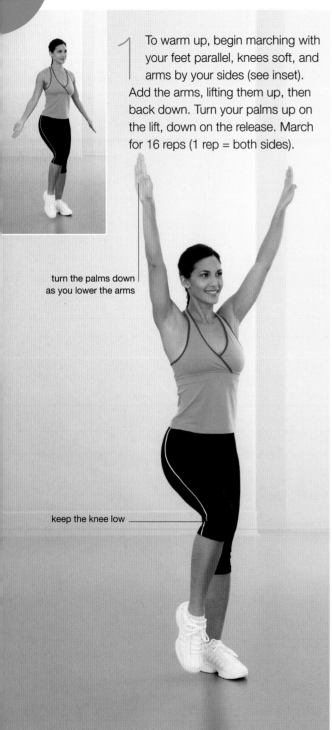

turn the palms down as you lower the arms

keep the knee low

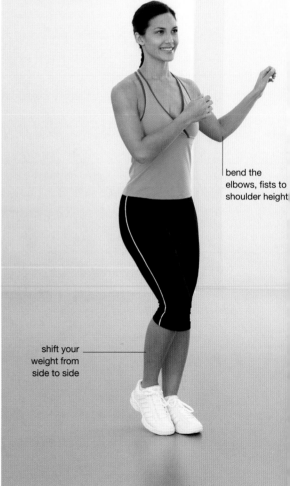

bend the elbows, fists to shoulder height

shift your weight from side to side

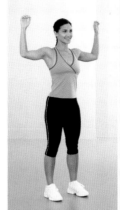

3 Step your feet apart, arms by your sides (see inset). Swing both arms to one side at shoulder height, coming up on the toes of the opposite foot. Circle your arms down to the other side and reach out with the tapping leg. Repeat, alternating sides for 8 reps.

4 With legs apart, raise the arms sideways to shoulder height. Bend elbows to 90 degrees, palms forwards (see inset). Keeping the back straight, bend one knee to hip height. Rotate your torso, bringing the opposite elbow towards the raised knee. Repeat, alternating sides for 8 reps.

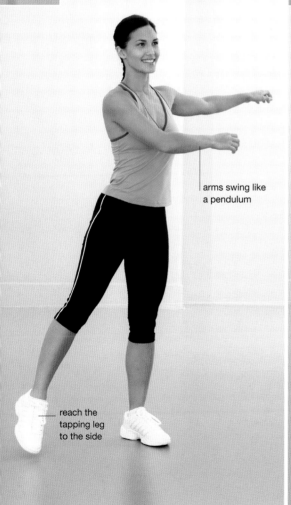

arms swing like a pendulum

reach the tapping leg to the side

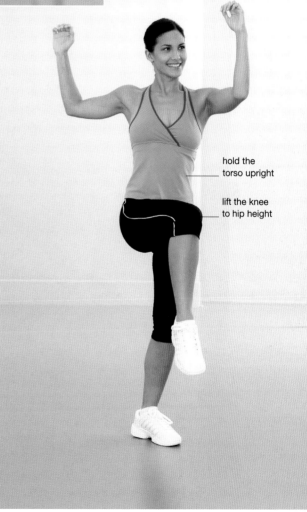

hold the torso upright

lift the knee to hip height

>> **hamstring curl/body sway**

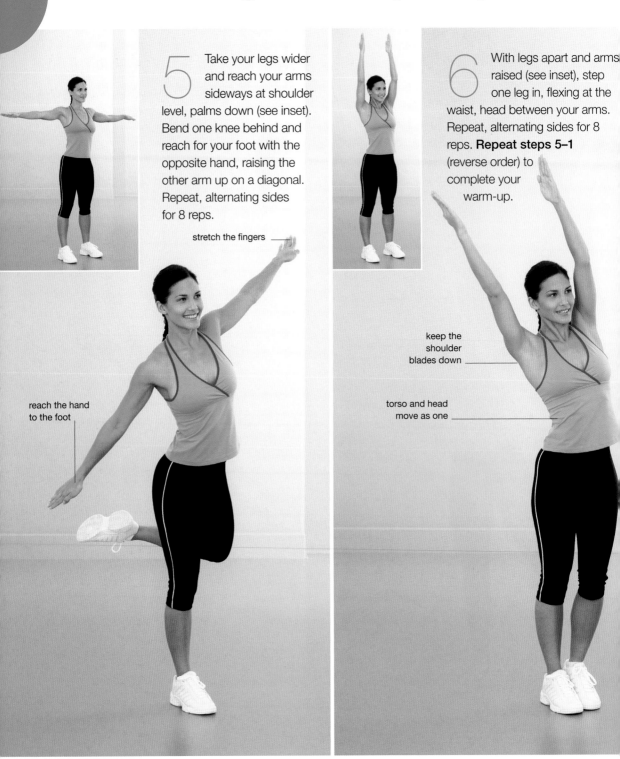

5 Take your legs wider and reach your arms sideways at shoulder level, palms down (see inset). Bend one knee behind and reach for your foot with the opposite hand, raising the other arm up on a diagonal. Repeat, alternating sides for 8 reps.

stretch the fingers

reach the hand to the foot

6 With legs apart and arms raised (see inset), step one leg in, flexing at the waist, head between your arms. Repeat, alternating sides for 8 reps. **Repeat steps 5–1** (reverse order) to complete your warm-up.

keep the shoulder blades down

torso and head move as one

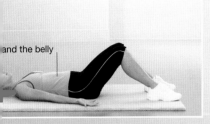

and the belly

7 Lie in neutral position, knees bent at 90 degrees, hip-width apart and feet flat on the floor. Rest your arms by your sides, palms up. Begin with a belly breath (see inset), then exhale forcefully, compress your abdomen and rotate your pelvis backwards, pressing your low back to the floor. Hold for a moment, then release. Repeat for 10 reps.

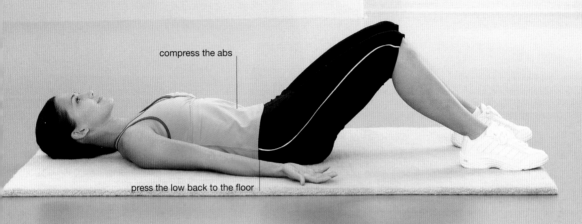

compress the abs

press the low back to the floor

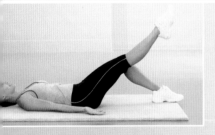

8 In neutral position, do a strong Pelvic Tilt and release halfway so your low back goes into its natural curve. Keep your abs tight to stabilize your pelvis in this position. Extend one leg to the height of the other knee (see inset). Inhale and slowly lower the leg towards the floor; exhale and return to start. Repeat 6 times, then change sides.

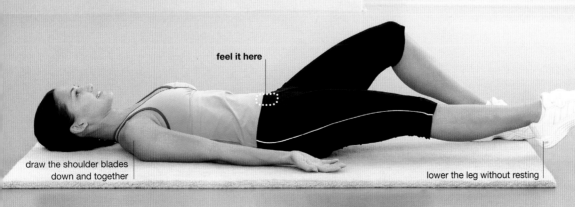

feel it here

draw the shoulder blades down and together

lower the leg without resting

>> 90–90/alternating kicks

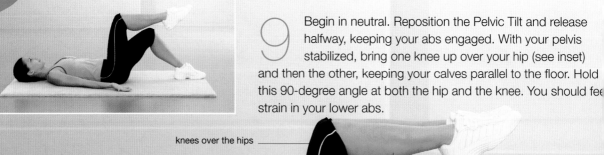

9 Begin in neutral. Reposition the Pelvic Tilt and release halfway, keeping your abs engaged. With your pelvis stabilized, bring one knee up over your hip (see inset) and then the other, keeping your calves parallel to the floor. Hold this 90-degree angle at both the hip and the knee. You should feel strain in your lower abs.

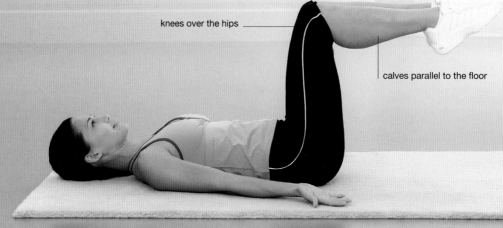

knees over the hips

calves parallel to the floor

10 From 90–90, bring one knee in over your chest and straighten the other leg, lowering it as close to the floor as possible without arching your back. Pause, then return to the start position and repeat, alternating legs for 5 reps. Hug your knees into your chest and rock from side to side.

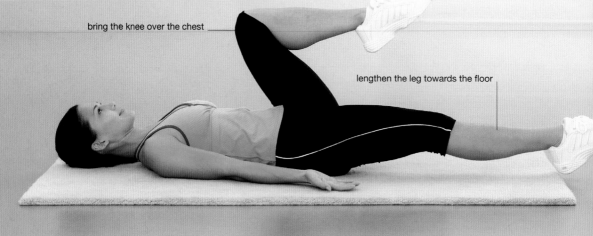

bring the knee over the chest

lengthen the leg towards the floor

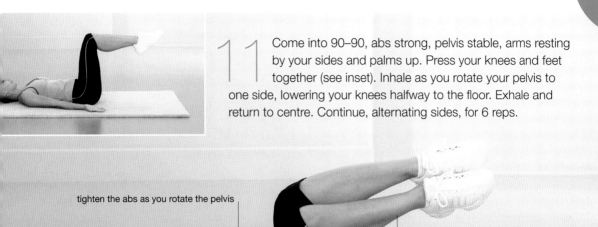

11 Come into 90–90, abs strong, pelvis stable, arms resting by your sides and palms up. Press your knees and feet together (see inset). Inhale as you rotate your pelvis to one side, lowering your knees halfway to the floor. Exhale and return to centre. Continue, alternating sides, for 6 reps.

tighten the abs as you rotate the pelvis

legs together, knees and ankles stacked

12 Bring your feet to the floor in neutral position, then rotate your knees to one side. Stretch your arms out to the sides at shoulder level, palms up. Rest, turning your head to the opposite side. Hold the position briefly and breathe, then change sides.

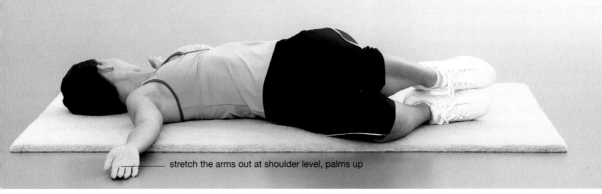

stretch the arms out at shoulder level, palms up

>> double-leg lowering

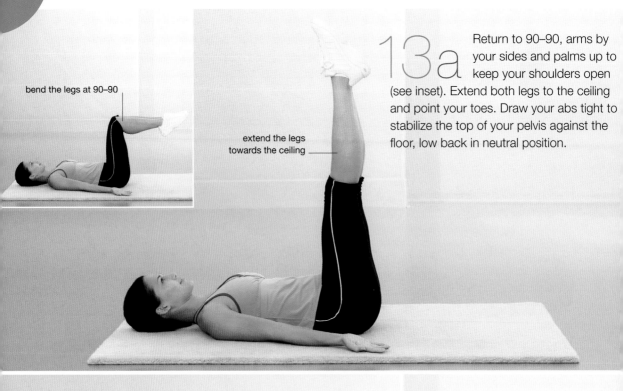

bend the legs at 90–90

extend the legs
towards the ceiling

13a

Return to 90–90, arms by
your sides and palms up to
keep your shoulders open
(see inset). Extend both legs to the ceiling
and point your toes. Draw your abs tight to
stabilize the top of your pelvis against the
floor, low back in neutral position.

13b

Exhale as you lower both legs towards the floor,
going as far as you can without arching your low
back. Keep pulling your abs in as you go. Inhale,
bend your knees in and return to start. Repeat 10 times. Hug your
knees in to rest.

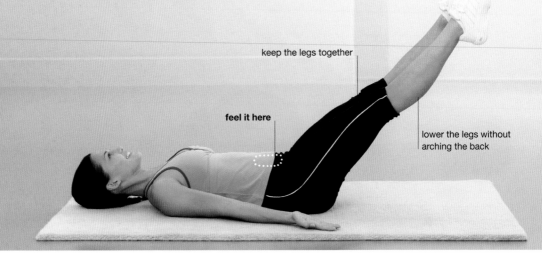

keep the legs together

feel it here

lower the legs without
arching the back

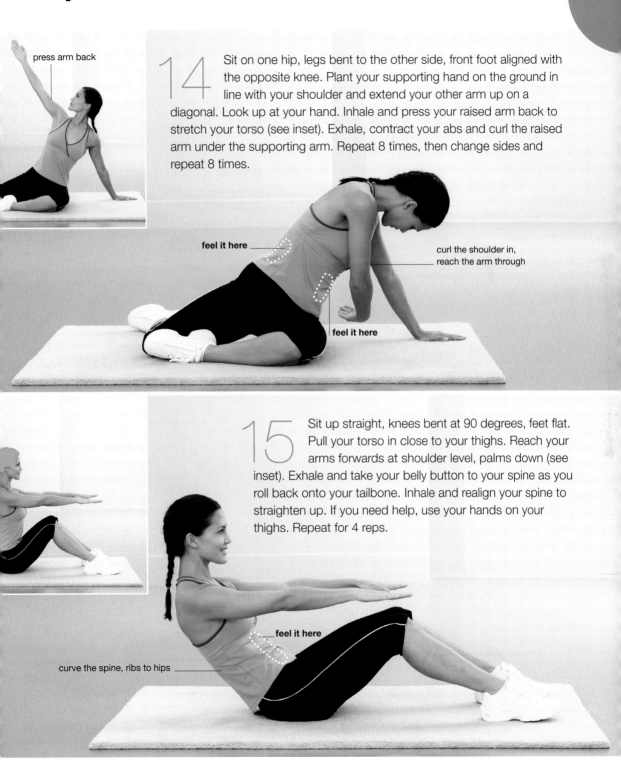

press arm back

14 Sit on one hip, legs bent to the other side, front foot aligned with the opposite knee. Plant your supporting hand on the ground in line with your shoulder and extend your other arm up on a diagonal. Look up at your hand. Inhale and press your raised arm back to stretch your torso (see inset). Exhale, contract your abs and curl the raised arm under the supporting arm. Repeat 8 times, then change sides and repeat 8 times.

feel it here

curl the shoulder in, reach the arm through

feel it here

15 Sit up straight, knees bent at 90 degrees, feet flat. Pull your torso in close to your thighs. Reach your arms forwards at shoulder level, palms down (see inset). Exhale and take your belly button to your spine as you roll back onto your tailbone. Inhale and realign your spine to straighten up. If you need help, use your hands on your thighs. Repeat for 4 reps.

feel it here

curve the spine, ribs to hips

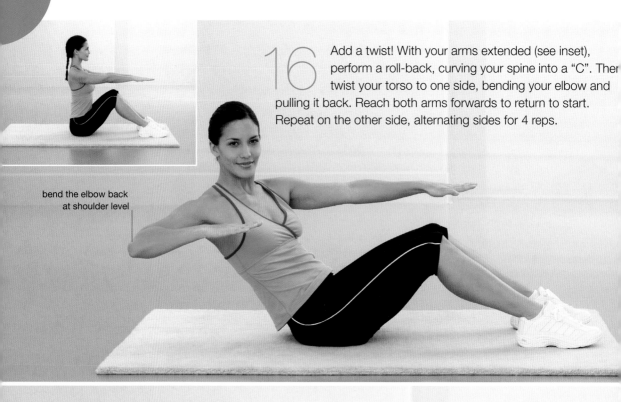

16 Add a twist! With your arms extended (see inset), perform a roll-back, curving your spine into a "C". Then twist your torso to one side, bending your elbow and pulling it back. Reach both arms forwards to return to start. Repeat on the other side, alternating sides for 4 reps.

bend the elbow back at shoulder level

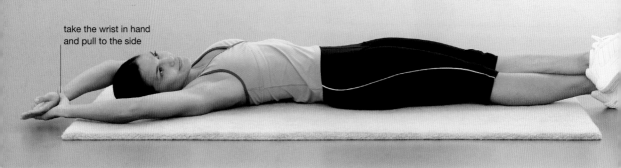

17 Holding onto your thighs, roll down to the floor and extend your arms and legs. Take a deep breath in and stretch out as far as you can. Exhale and relax. Cross one ankle over the other and take the wrist on the same side in your other hand. Pull to the opposite side, creating a stretch down one side of your body. Repeat on the other side.

take the wrist in hand and pull to the side

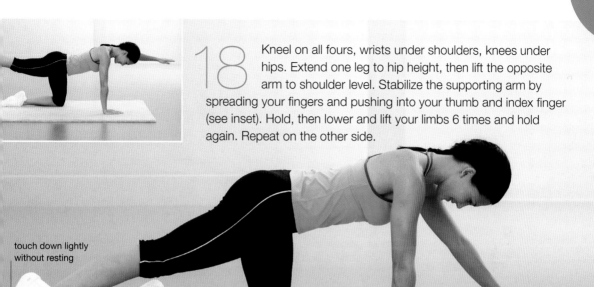

18 Kneel on all fours, wrists under shoulders, knees under hips. Extend one leg to hip height, then lift the opposite arm to shoulder level. Stabilize the supporting arm by spreading your fingers and pushing into your thumb and index finger (see inset). Hold, then lower and lift your limbs 6 times and hold again. Repeat on the other side.

touch down lightly without resting

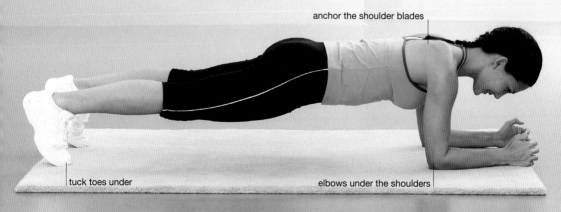

19 From the kneeling position, take your hands forwards and place your forearms on the floor, elbows directly under your shoulders. Take your knees back and drop your hips, creating a straight line from shoulder to knee. Pull your abs tight and anchor your shoulder blades (see inset). Hold, then straighten your legs and come onto your toes in the Full Forearm Plank position. Hold.

anchor the shoulder blades

tuck toes under   elbows under the shoulders

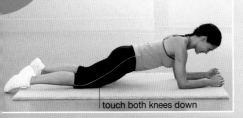

touch both knees down

20 From the Full Plank, lower both knees simultaneously 4 times (see inset). Then lower one knee at a time, alternating sides for 4 reps. If you are fatiguing, just try to hold the Forearm Plank from the knees. Breathe naturally throughout.

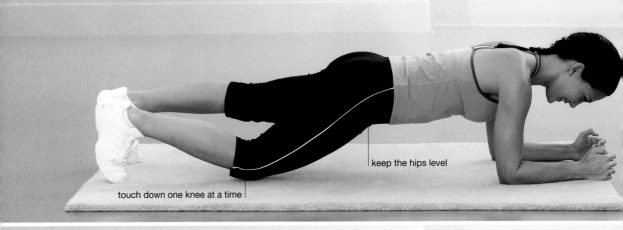

keep the hips level

touch down one knee at a time

21 Sit back into Child's Pose, with your hips to your heels and your forehead to the floor. Stretch your arms forwards. Take a few seconds to rest in this position and refresh yourself. Breathe deeply, releasing tension from your muscles with every exhale.

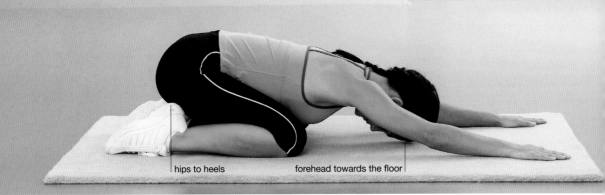

hips to heels

forehead towards the floor

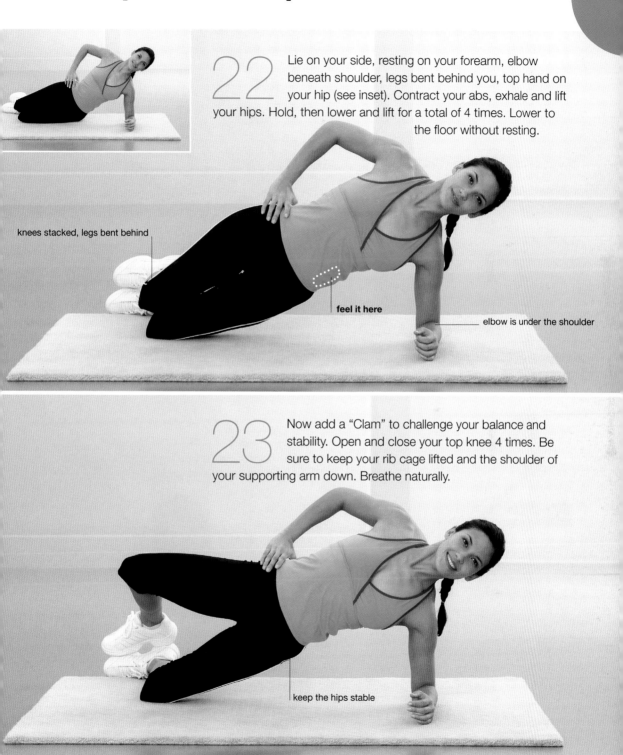

22 Lie on your side, resting on your forearm, elbow beneath shoulder, legs bent behind you, top hand on your hip (see inset). Contract your abs, exhale and lift your hips. Hold, then lower and lift for a total of 4 times. Lower to the floor without resting.

knees stacked, legs bent behind

feel it here

elbow is under the shoulder

23 Now add a "Clam" to challenge your balance and stability. Open and close your top knee 4 times. Be sure to keep your rib cage lifted and the shoulder of your supporting arm down. Breathe naturally.

keep the hips stable

24 Lower your hips to the floor and sit up. Separating your legs, bend your knees to the side and reach your opposite arm overhead, palm down. Stretch out the muscles that you just worked, especially the obliques and then repeat steps 22–24 on the other side.

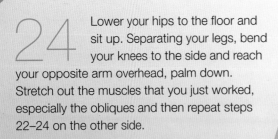

keep the shoulder blade down

weight on the front hip

25 Sit tall and open your legs in a wide "V" (see inset). Lean forwards from your hips with your spine straight and reach your arms to centre. Keeping both hips planted evenly on the floor, lift your spine, then turn your torso to face one leg and hold. Pass through centre and repeat on the other side.

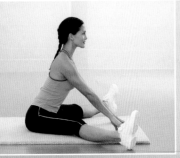

spine straight

hips firmly planted

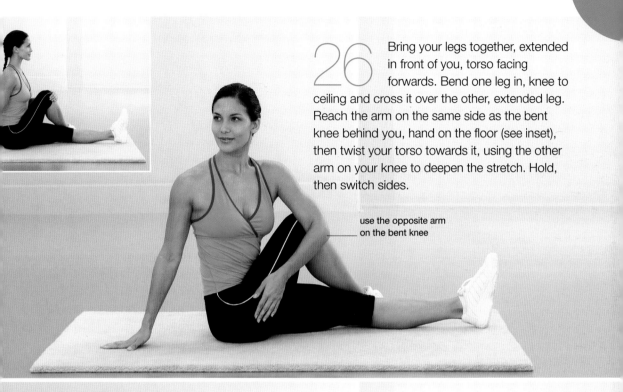

26 Bring your legs together, extended in front of you, torso facing forwards. Bend one leg in, knee to ceiling and cross it over the other, extended leg. Reach the arm on the same side as the bent knee behind you, hand on the floor (see inset), then twist your torso towards it, using the other arm on your knee to deepen the stretch. Hold, then switch sides.

use the opposite arm
on the bent knee

27 Turn your torso back to centre. Straighten your spine, lift up and out of the low back and then reach your head forwards. Relax over your knees, breathing deeply.

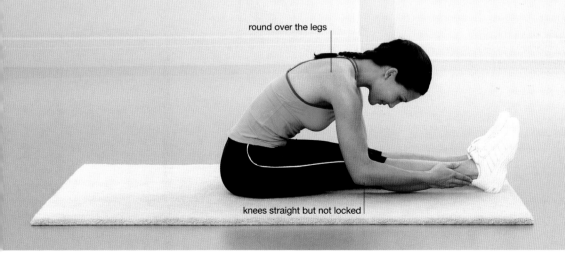

round over the legs

knees straight but not locked

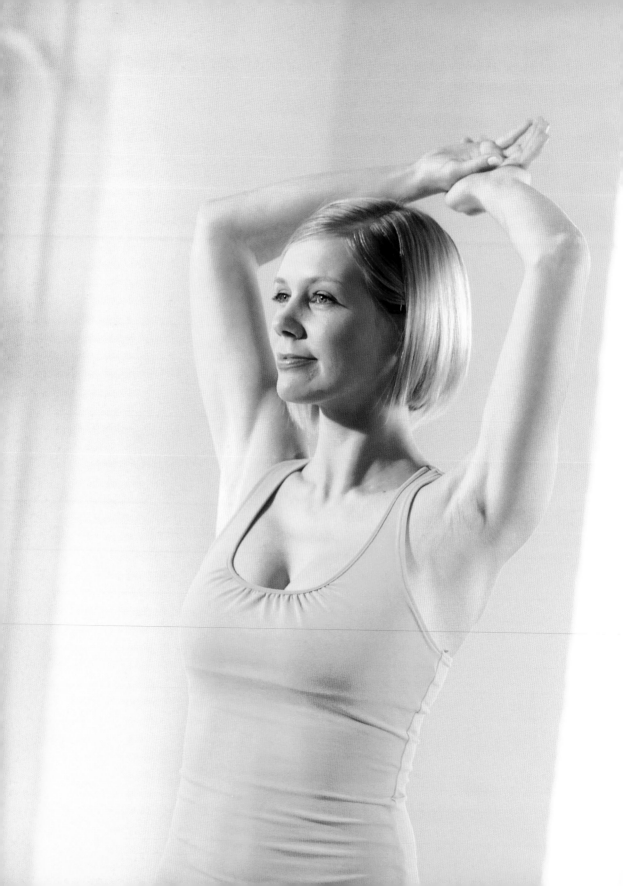

>> **15** minute

better back
workout

Suzanne Martin P.T., D.P.T.

>> **the parts of** the back

Take a moment at this point to review the four different parts of the back.

Each has a different role to play in enabling us to perform our everyday tasks.

Getting a clear idea of the four main sections of your back will help you to

make your exercises more effective. Look in the mirror and follow along.

The "back" is technically the "spine" and is made up of several parts. Looking from the side, it makes a long S-curve. The spine has four main curves: the cervical, the thoracic, the lumbar and the fused sacral/coccyx. The curves are not present at birth and only begin to develop when an infant achieves vertical standing and at toddler stage when he or she begins to walk. The downward press of gravity shapes the spine and gives each curve an all-important role in maintaining the health of the back and producing bipedal stance.

The cervical spine
The cervical spine or upper neck can be felt at your hairline, just at the base of the skull. It is responsible for tipping the chin upwards and downwards. The upper part of the cervical spine also contains the muscles responsible for eye motions. If you keep your fingertips at the base and dart your eyes back and forth, you'll detect the motions of these fine muscles.

The lower cervical spine is convex-shaped. You can usually feel the prominent southernmost vertebra as it meets the shoulders. The neck has the greatest amount of range of motion of the spine. It can create a telescoping effect and can swivel to almost look completely behind you.

The thoracic spine
This has a concave shape and is connected with the rib cage. You can trace the prominent spinous processes, the visible bumps of the spine, by

> ## >> **the four main** parts of the back
>
> - **The cervical spine**, or "neck", has seven vertebrae and extends from the base of the skull to the shoulders.
> - **The thoracic spine**, comprising the upper and mid-back, has 12 vertebrae and extends from the shoulders to the waist.
> - **The lumbar spine**, or "lower back", has five vertebrae. This vulnerable section forms the waist and has no bony support.
> - **The sacral section** contains the four fused vertebrae of the sacrum with the vestigial tail, the coccyx, at its end.

running your thumbs from your shoulders down to the top of your waist. It is chronically stiff since it's girdled by the rib cage, so developing mobility in the thoracic spine requires patience.

The lumbar spine
Put your hands around your waist to find the lumbar spine. This part of the spine is particularly vulnerable because it's balancing the weight of the trunk against the unwieldy weighty legs. What's special about the lumbar spine is its springboard effect on the spine. Its convex shape allows the impact against the ground to dissipate as you step.

The back is not a single entity but is actually made up of four main sections. The exercises in *Better Back Workout* will help you strengthen each of them.

The curves make an S-shape that gives the back resilience. Preserving those curves is all-important if you want a pain-free back!

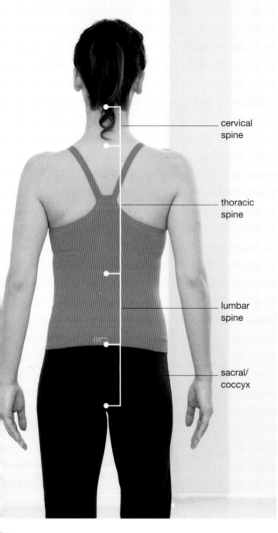

cervical spine

thoracic spine

lumbar spine

sacral/coccyx

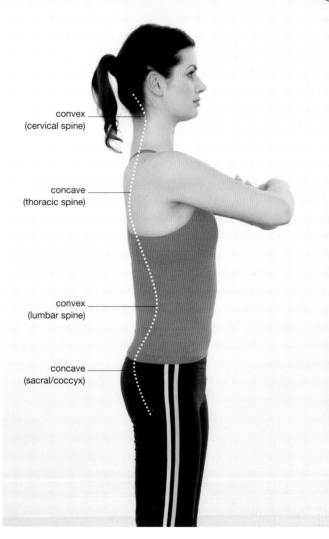

convex (cervical spine)

concave (thoracic spine)

convex (lumbar spine)

concave (sacral/coccyx)

The sacrum

Finally, place your hands on your hip bones, fingers facing forwards, and your thumbs will end up on top of the fused vertebrae of the sacrum. Very large forces converge here – at the sacroiliac joints – the place where the lumbar spine and the sacrum meet. That means that this area is extremely vulnerable and requires careful positioning and handling if you are to avoid injury. At the bottom of this fusion lies the coccyx, or tailbone.

The discs

These are pieces of cartilage that lie between the vertebrae. Think of them as being like doughnuts, with a soft centre and a hard exterior. They provide cushioning in between the vertebrae but, even more importantly, they give range to the spine so it can bend and twist as required. Protecting the spine means protecting these all-important discs. And that is achieved by strengthening the back and by learning posture control.

>> **posture** and the back

Posture is important both to the strength of your back and to how you appear. It can make you look dumpy, tired and old, or together, confident and lithe. Fortunately, posture is not all down to your genetic inheritance. There is much you can do to improve it and prevent gravity from winning out.

The slump

This posture pushes the head forwards out of line, rounds the shoulders and leads to a slouched pelvis. Besides being aesthetically unappealing, it places enormous strain on the discs.

The sway back

Catwalk models perform the sway to make themselves appear "cool". The sway-back posture makes the shoulders lean and compresses the lower spine while reversing the thoracic area. In a nutshell – stand up straight!

Hyperlordosis

This is an exaggerated curve of the lumbar spine. It weakens the springboard effect provided by the lower back to the rest of the spine. It also shortens the stabilizing muscles of the pelvis. It's not only pregnant women and those with apple-body types who fall into this category. Athletic people tend to get tight hips that can throw them into this posture.

Below left to right The slump, the sway back and hyperlordosis are three typical bad postures. Each will cause problems for the body sooner or later.

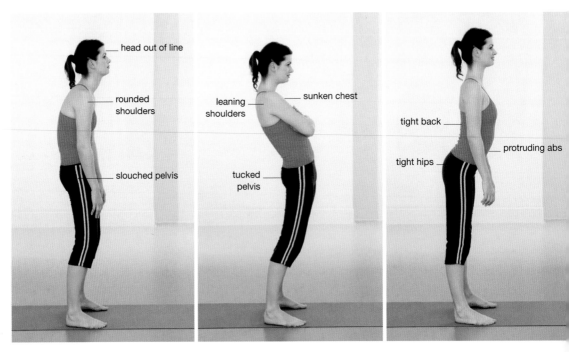

head out of line

rounded shoulders

slouched pelvis

leaning shoulders

sunken chest

tucked pelvis

tight back

protruding abs

tight hips

See the difference between bad and good posture. On the left, bad posture is sure to mean aches and pains. On the right, good posture looks healthy and is healthy.

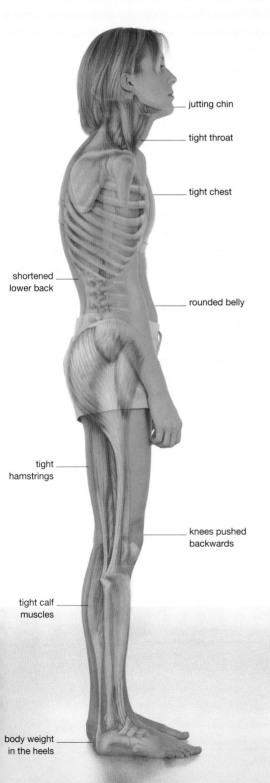

jutting chin

tight throat

tight chest

shortened lower back

rounded belly

tight hamstrings

knees pushed backwards

tight calf muscles

body weight in the heels

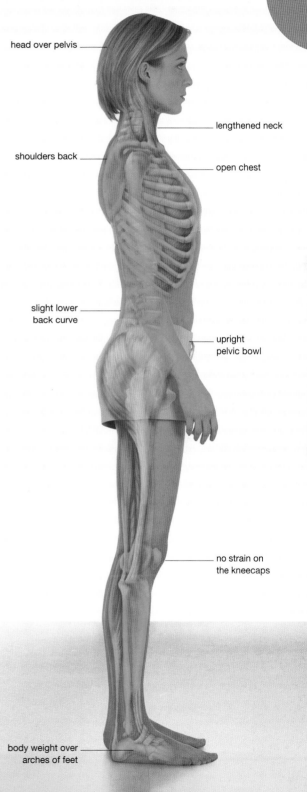

head over pelvis

lengthened neck

shoulders back

open chest

slight lower back curve

upright pelvic bowl

no strain on the kneecaps

body weight over arches of feet

>> **protecting** the back

The back requires extra protection because it has so many interconnecting parts. If one part gets injured, so do all the others. There are certain moves we all perform every day that involve the back. Performing them correctly, as shown here, can go a long way towards protecting the spine.

First position parallel means bringing your feet straight under your pelvis. It is the healthiest position to adopt for your legs and gives the greatest support for your spine.

"Butt-ski, out-ski" is the humorous name for this bending position (below right). It is ergonomically best for the discs of your lower back, which can be severely and irreparably damaged when bending, and particularly when lifting and twisting at the same time. It's really simple; just think of bending from your hips, sticking your bottom out and using your legs to take the strain as you stand up.

The log roll is particularly helpful, especially for getting in and out of bed or up and down from lying on the floor. It's an excellent strategy when your back is painful and sore. It's shown on the opposite page in four simple steps.

Below left For first position parallel take your feet about 10cm (4in) apart, with your second toe lining up with your kneecap and with the point midway on your groin line.

Below When you are bending, bend at your hips and keep your back straight. For lifting, always think "butt-ski, out-ski" (stick your bottom out) and lift with your legs.

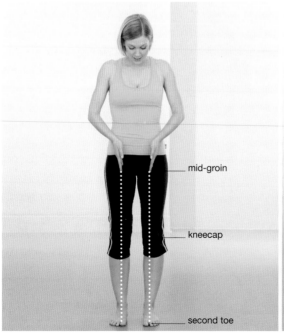

mid-groin

kneecap

second toe

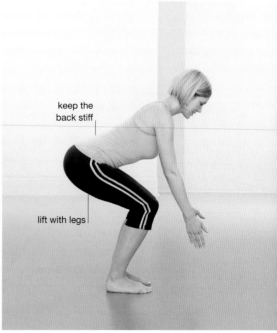

keep the back stiff

lift with legs

1 First, while lying on your back, tighten your waist and abdomen. Next, keep your back stiff just as in the "butt-ski, out-ski" position (see opposite) and brace your bent legs.

2 Roll onto your side as a unit with your shoulders and hips; don't twist at your waist. Keep your legs together. When getting out of bed, let your feet go over the side.

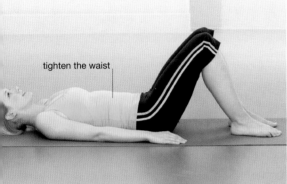

tighten the waist

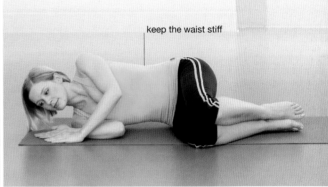

keep the waist stiff

3 Next, use your arms, not your back, to push yourself up to sitting. When getting out of bed, let your feet dangle over the edge as soon as possible.

4 Sit tall, lift your breastbone and bring your head over your pelvis. Press down on your sitting bones and straighten up through your spine. Feel as if your spine is being sucked up through a straw towards your head.

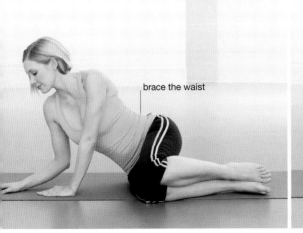

brace the waist

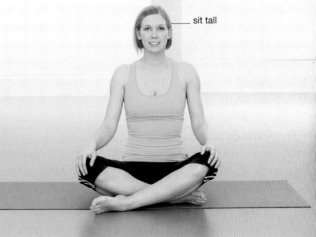

sit tall

15 minute

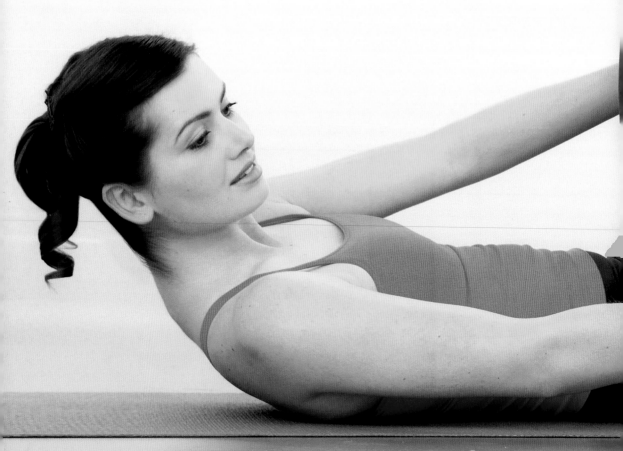

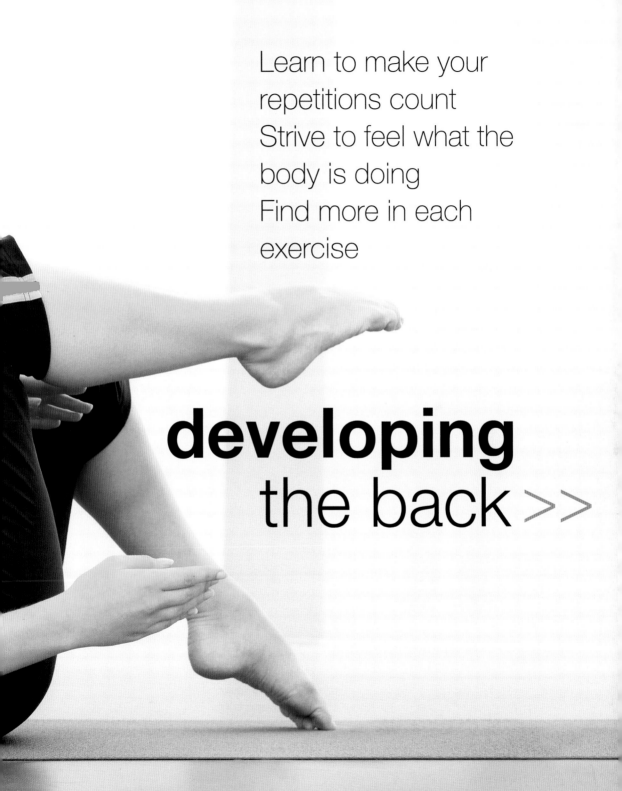

Learn to make your
repetitions count
Strive to feel what the
body is doing
Find more in each
exercise

developing
the back >>

>> upper rolls

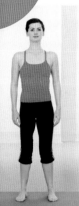

1 Stand tall with your feet about shoulder-width apart (see inset). Lift up the abdominals upward from the pubic bone toward the navel. Open your chest and take your head over your pelvis. Breathe in and out as you count to 8 while slowly rolling your shoulders backwards.

2 Hold your waist firm. Fold your elbows and bring your hands to your shoulders. Make full, yet comfortable circles with your elbows about 5 times. Then reverse the direction for 5 more circles.

roll the
shoulders
backwards

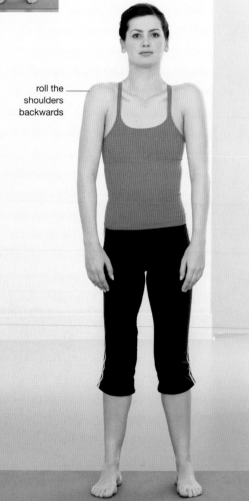

hold the
waist firm

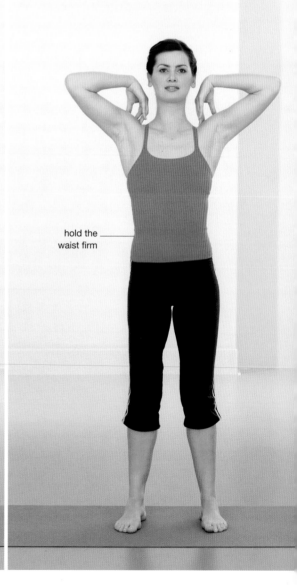

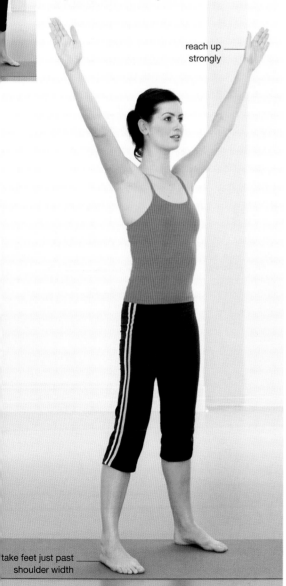

3 Place your feet just past shoulder-width apart (see inset). Reach your arms up sideways with your palms facing forwards. Reach up and wide. Open your mouth and eyes.

reach up strongly

take feet just past shoulder width

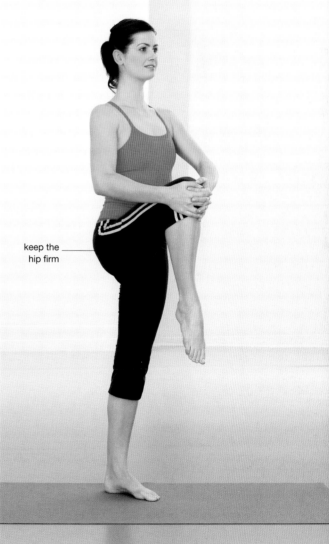

4 Balance on your left leg, then exhale and squeeze your right knee to your waist. Find your balance, then return to stand on both feet with your arms reaching upwards. Now balance on your right leg and squeeze your left knee to your waist. Repeat this alternation from right to left for 3 more sets.

keep the hip firm

>> knee circles

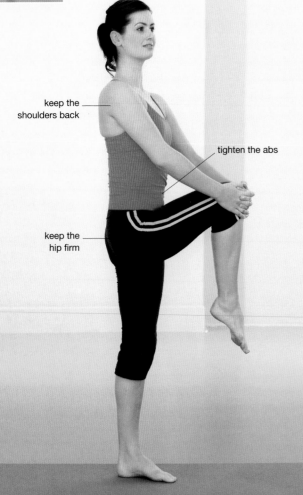

5 Stand on your left leg and be aware of your balance. Tighten your abs and hold your right knee steady to your waist with both hands (see inset). Anchor your shoulders back. Hold onto a piece of furniture if you can't manage to balance. Circle your knee 3 times.

6 Exhale and bow your head to your right knee and feel the stretch in your back. Release. Stand on your right leg and repeat the balance and circles. End with a bow to your left knee.

keep the
shoulders back

tighten the abs

keep the
hip firm

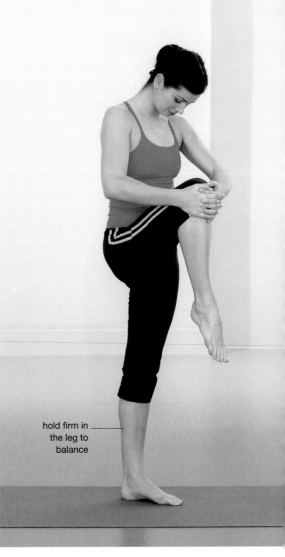

hold firm in
the leg to
balance

>> side stretch 1

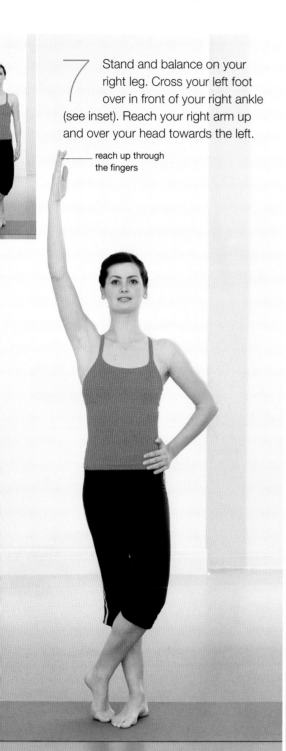

7 Stand and balance on your right leg. Cross your left foot over in front of your right ankle (see inset). Reach your right arm up and over your head towards the left.

reach up through the fingers

8 Zip up the tight jeans and firmly push your left hand in a horizontal motion against your left hip so you bend to the left. Breathe in and out 4 times. Come back to centre. Uncross your leg and repeat to stretch your left side the same way.

feel it here

hold the abs

tuck the hip in

>> squat stretch

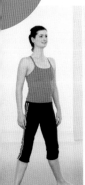

9 Open your legs past shoulder width and turn your toes slightly outwards (see inset). Hold your waist tight, and firm your bottom as you bend straight down inside your legs to place your hands on top of your knees.

10 Lift your pelvis and lengthen your spine. Inhale, press your right hand against your right knee, then exhale and turn your shoulders to look diagonally up and to your left. Breathe in and out 3 times. Stand up, then repeat the stretch to the other side.

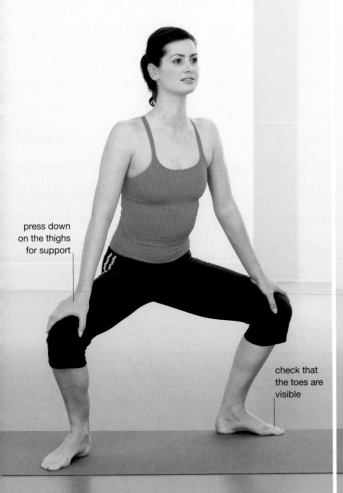

press down on the thighs for support

check that the toes are visible

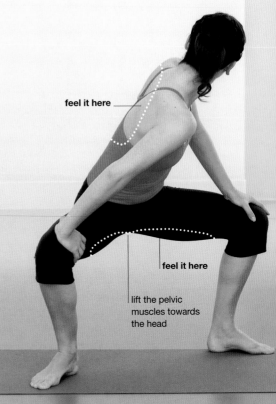

feel it here

feel it here

lift the pelvic muscles towards the head

>> toe touches

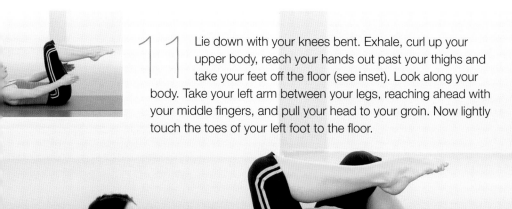

11 Lie down with your knees bent. Exhale, curl up your upper body, reach your hands out past your thighs and take your feet off the floor (see inset). Look along your body. Take your left arm between your legs, reaching ahead with your middle fingers, and pull your head to your groin. Now lightly touch the toes of your left foot to the floor.

press the lower back into the floor

strongly reach the middle fingers out parallel to the floor

12 Simultaneously touch your right foot to the floor as you raise your left. Alternate toe touches for 16 repetitions. Place your right arm between your legs and alternate toe touches 16 more times. To end, hold both legs and arms up and increase the pull of your middle fingers.

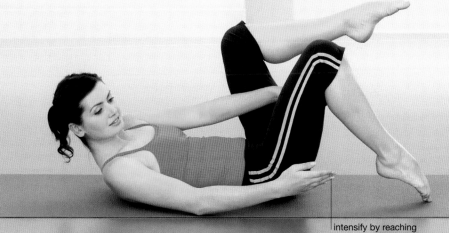

intensify by reaching harder with the fingers

>> side bends

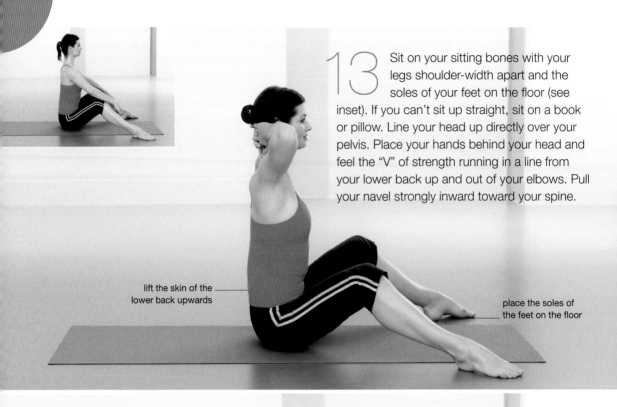

13 Sit on your sitting bones with your legs shoulder-width apart and the soles of your feet on the floor (see inset). If you can't sit up straight, sit on a book or pillow. Line your head up directly over your pelvis. Place your hands behind your head and feel the "V" of strength running in a line from your lower back up and out of your elbows. Pull your navel strongly inward toward your spine.

lift the skin of the lower back upwards

place the soles of the feet on the floor

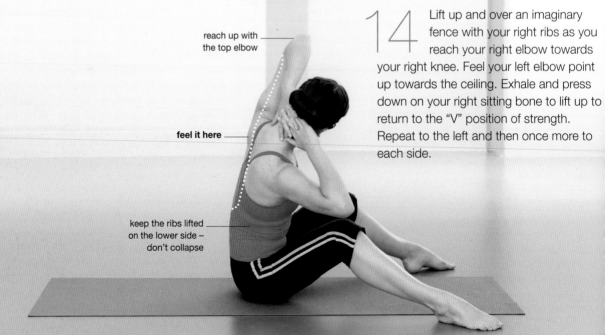

reach up with the top elbow

14 Lift up and over an imaginary fence with your right ribs as you reach your right elbow towards your right knee. Feel your left elbow point up towards the ceiling. Exhale and press down on your right sitting bone to lift up to return to the "V" position of strength. Repeat to the left and then once more to each side.

feel it here

keep the ribs lifted on the lower side – don't collapse

>> overhead squeeze

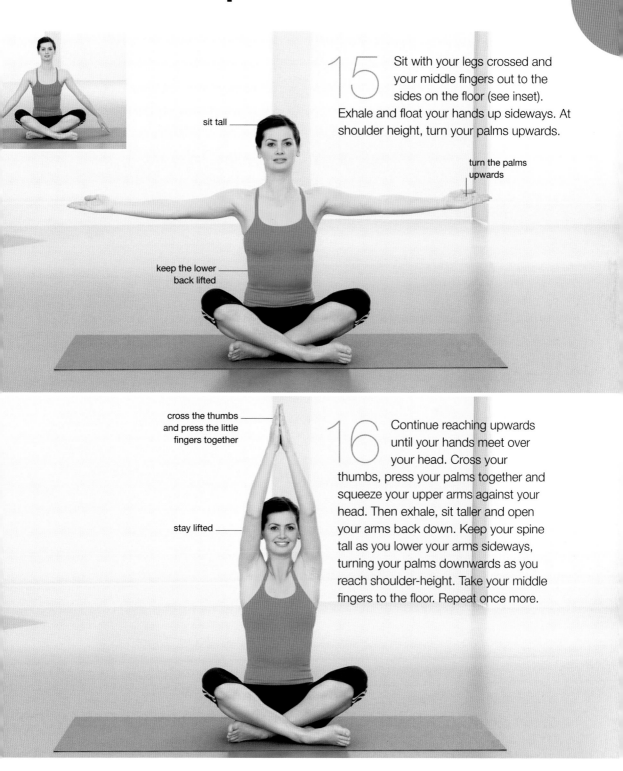

sit tall

keep the lower
back lifted

turn the palms
upwards

15 Sit with your legs crossed and your middle fingers out to the sides on the floor (see inset). Exhale and float your hands up sideways. At shoulder height, turn your palms upwards.

cross the thumbs
and press the little
fingers together

stay lifted

16 Continue reaching upwards until your hands meet over your head. Cross your thumbs, press your palms together and squeeze your upper arms against your head. Then exhale, sit taller and open your arms back down. Keep your spine tall as you lower your arms sideways, turning your palms downwards as you reach shoulder-height. Take your middle fingers to the floor. Repeat once more.

>> temple

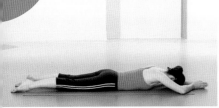

17 Lie on your front. Feel the imaginary swimming pool water lift your abs off the floor. Reach your hands above your head on the floor, with elbows bent and palms together (see inset). Knit your ribs together to engage your solar plexus. Tuck your toes under to make little stands. Tighten the muscles in the hips and back of the thighs.

pull the tailbone
towards the heels

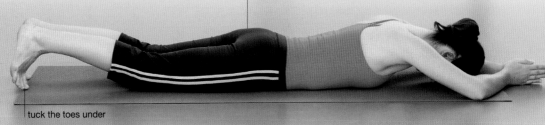

tuck the toes under

18 Inhale, then exhale as you levitate your hands and forearms off the floor, while at the same time straightening your knees so they come off the floor as well. Stay as you take a couple of breaths, then exhale and lower. Relax and then repeat the sequence.

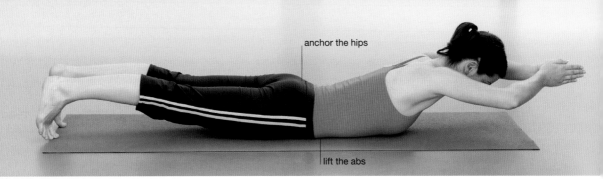

anchor the hips

lift the abs

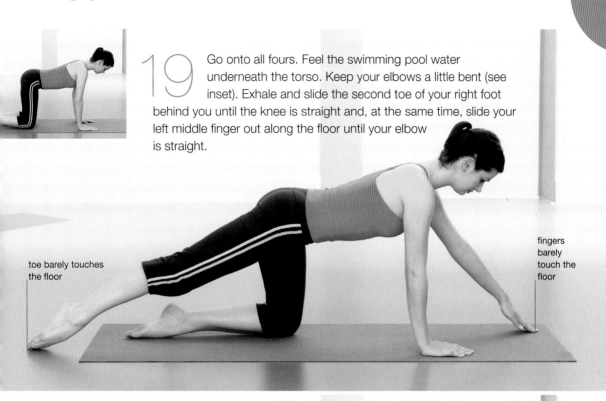

19 Go onto all fours. Feel the swimming pool water underneath the torso. Keep your elbows a little bent (see inset). Exhale and slide the second toe of your right foot behind you until the knee is straight and, at the same time, slide your left middle finger out along the floor until your elbow is straight.

toe barely touches the floor

fingers barely touch the floor

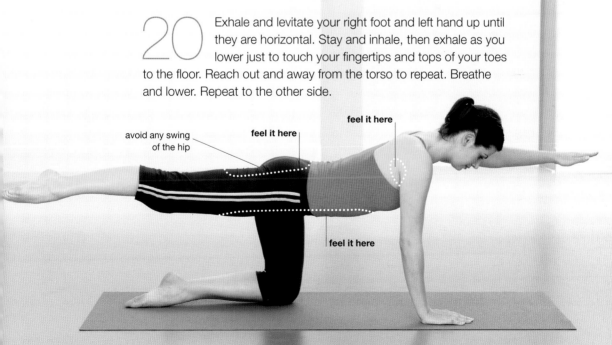

20 Exhale and levitate your right foot and left hand up until they are horizontal. Stay and inhale, then exhale as you lower just to touch your fingertips and tops of your toes to the floor. Reach out and away from the torso to repeat. Breathe and lower. Repeat to the other side.

feel it here

avoid any swing of the hip

feel it here

feel it here

feel it here

>> **plank push-up**

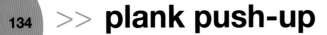

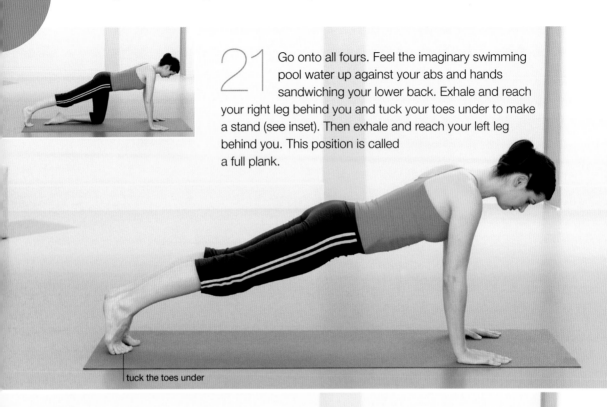

21 Go onto all fours. Feel the imaginary swimming pool water up against your abs and hands sandwiching your lower back. Exhale and reach your right leg behind you and tuck your toes under to make a stand (see inset). Then exhale and reach your left leg behind you. This position is called a full plank.

tuck the toes under

22 Inhale, bend the elbows and lower yourself in push-up style. Make smile lines. Exhale and stay, then inhale, exhale and come back up. Feel as if your abs have lifted you. Break at one hip and then the other to return to all fours. Repeat once more.

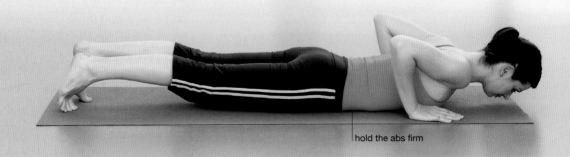

hold the abs firm

>> angel wings

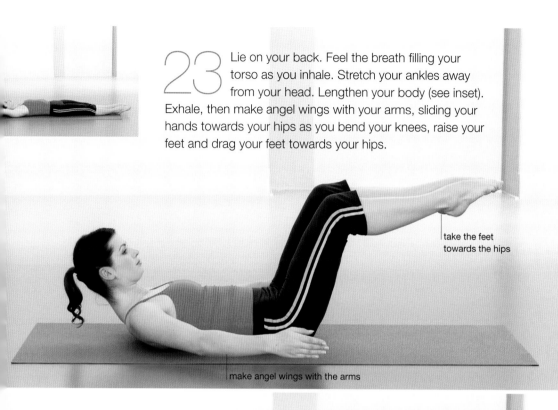

23 Lie on your back. Feel the breath filling your torso as you inhale. Stretch your ankles away from your head. Lengthen your body (see inset). Exhale, then make angel wings with your arms, sliding your hands towards your hips as you bend your knees, raise your feet and drag your feet towards your hips.

take the feet towards the hips

make angel wings with the arms

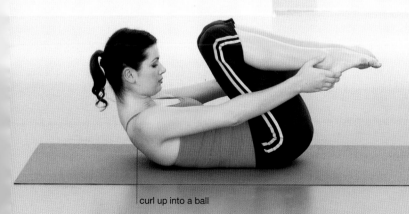

24 Reach to grab your heels, curling your body up into a little ball. Then inhale, lengthen your hips and legs down onto the floor again and repeat 3 more times. Hold and intensify the last curl, tightening your abs, then relax to the floor.

curl up into a ball

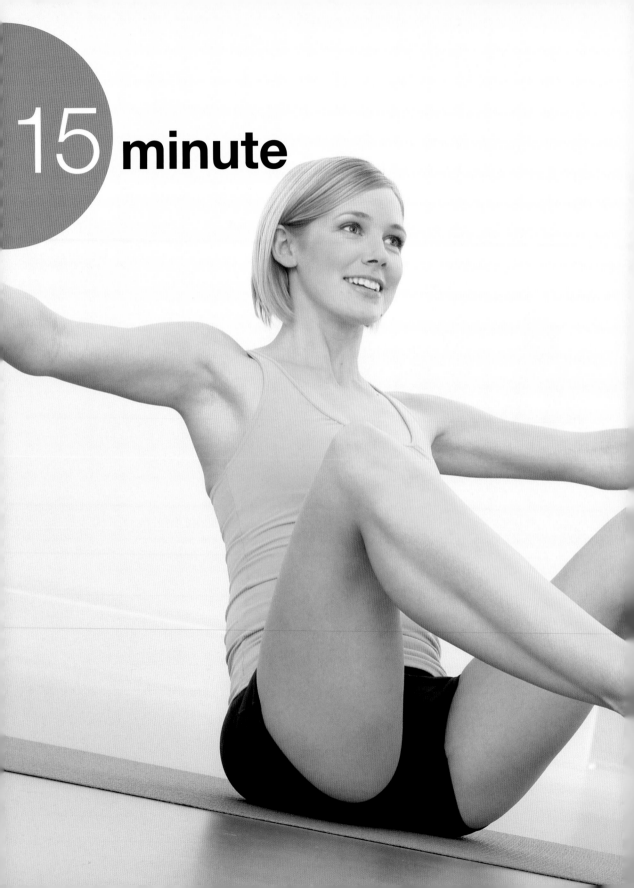

15 minute

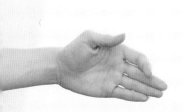

Accentuate the
changing rhythms
Notice your breath
Oxygen is key

revitalizing
the back >>

>> arm swing

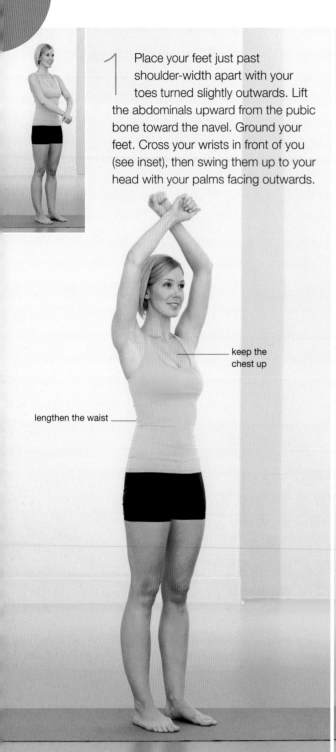

1 Place your feet just past shoulder-width apart with your toes turned slightly outwards. Lift the abdominals upward from the pubic bone toward the navel. Ground your feet. Cross your wrists in front of you (see inset), then swing them up to your head with your palms facing outwards.

keep the chest up

lengthen the waist

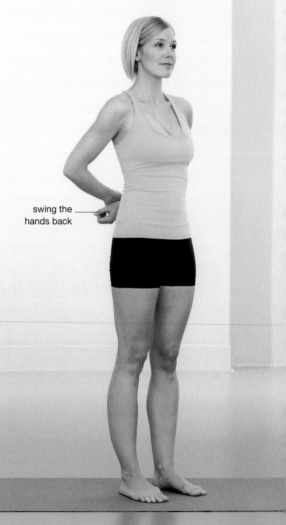

2 Swing your hands back and behind your hips so they touch together. Rhythmically swing your arms up and back using this motion 7 more times.

swing the hands back

3 Stand tall with your hands on your hips (see inset). Balance on your right leg, using a hand on a piece of furniture to support you if you need. Hold your hip firm on your right leg. Keep your chest up. Swing your left foot in front, as if you were wiping your foot on the ground.

4 Then swing your left foot down and back. Repeat this forwards and backwards motion easily and rhythmically 7 more times. Find your balance on your left leg and repeat, swinging your right leg.

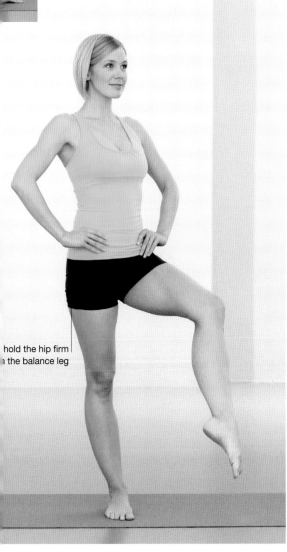

hold the hip firm on the balance leg

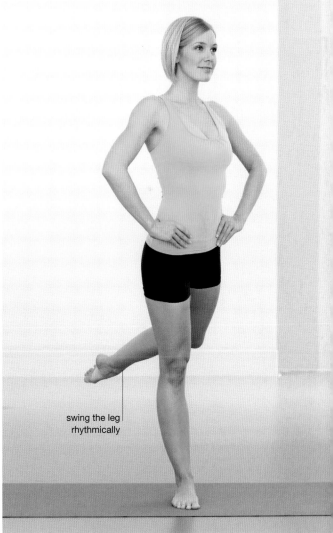

swing the leg rhythmically

>> tread in place

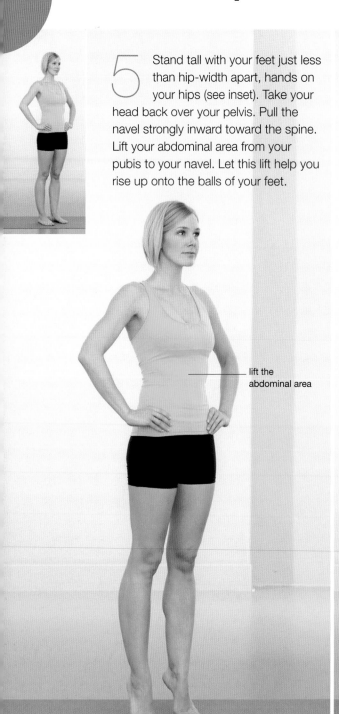

5 Stand tall with your feet just less than hip-width apart, hands on your hips (see inset). Take your head back over your pelvis. Pull the navel strongly inward toward the spine. Lift your abdominal area from your pubis to your navel. Let this lift help you rise up onto the balls of your feet.

lift the
abdominal area

6 Reach your head upwards as you lower your right heel, then rise up on the balls of your feet and lower your left heel. Repeat this treading motion 32 times.

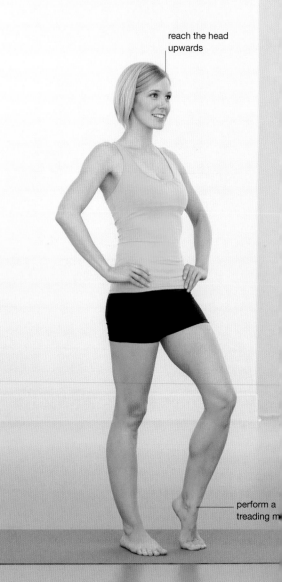

reach the head
upwards

perform a
treading m

>> tapping chest

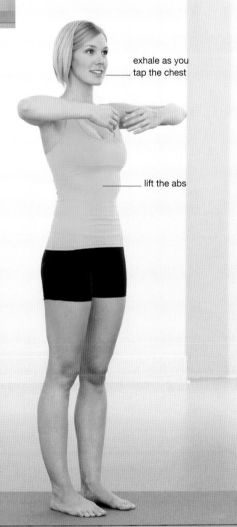

7 Stand tall with your feet just less than hip-width apart. Take your head back over your pelvis, pull your navel to your spine, lift your abdominals. Bring both hands to your breastbone (see inset). Gently tap your fingers on your breastbone as you exhale, saying "ha, ha, ha, ha" as you tap.

exhale as you tap the chest

lift the abs

8 Now inhale as you open your arms, making two big rainbow shapes up and out to the sides. Take your hands back to your breastbone and repeat the motion 4 more times, alternating the exhalation "ha's" with the inhalation rainbow shapes.

feel it here

feel it here

feel it here

revitalizing the back >>

>> side stretch 2

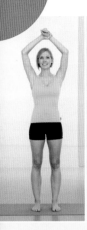

9 Stand with your arms above your head and your feet about hip-width apart (see inset). Anchor your left foot downwards as you grasp your left wrist with your right hand. Elongate and pull your wrist upwards.

10 Inhale as you lift up, to the right, as though you were leaning over a fence. Stay, exhale, lengthen. Then inhale, stay, then exhale and anchor the your foot again as you stretch back up to vertical, lengthening your waistline. Take your arms down. Repeat to the other side.

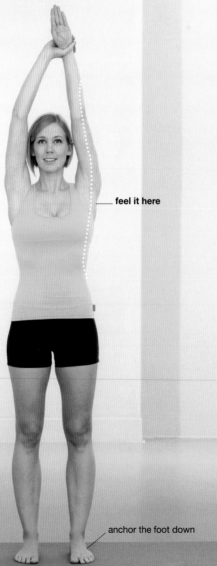

feel it here

anchor the foot down

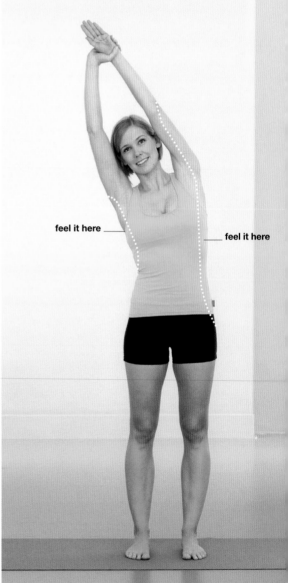

feel it here

feel it here

>> **stroke the cat**

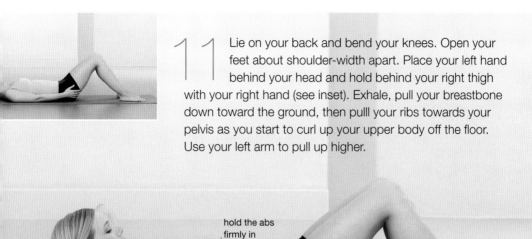

11 Lie on your back and bend your knees. Open your feet about shoulder-width apart. Place your left hand behind your head and hold behind your right thigh with your right hand (see inset). Exhale, pull your breastbone down toward the ground, then pulll your ribs towards your pelvis as you start to curl up your upper body off the floor. Use your left arm to pull up higher.

hold the abs
firmly in

press the lower back
against the floor

12 Now stroke the right thigh from bottom to top with the right hand, as if you were stroking a cat. Reach out past your knee with your middle finger. Stroke 6 times, then intensify the last stroke. Lower your upper body to the floor, then change arms to repeat, using your left hand and stroking your left thigh 6 times.

reach past the knees
with the middle finger

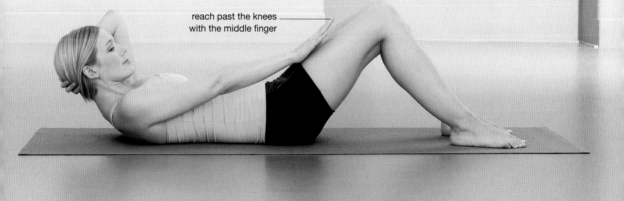

>> leg circles

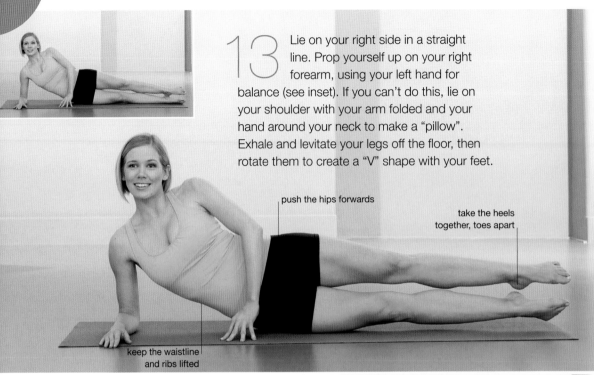

13 Lie on your right side in a straight line. Prop yourself up on your right forearm, using your left hand for balance (see inset). If you can't do this, lie on your shoulder with your arm folded and your hand around your neck to make a "pillow". Exhale and levitate your legs off the floor, then rotate them to create a "V" shape with your feet.

push the hips forwards

take the heels together, toes apart

keep the waistline and ribs lifted

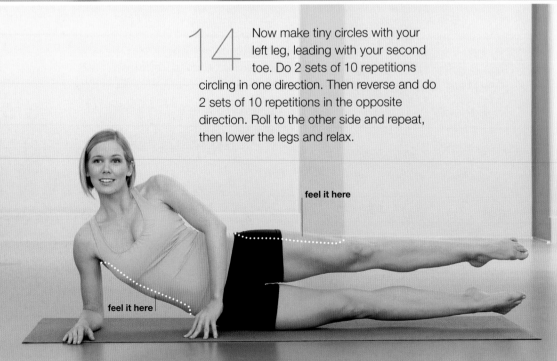

14 Now make tiny circles with your left leg, leading with your second toe. Do 2 sets of 10 repetitions circling in one direction. Then reverse and do 2 sets of 10 repetitions in the opposite direction. Roll to the other side and repeat, then lower the legs and relax.

feel it here

feel it here

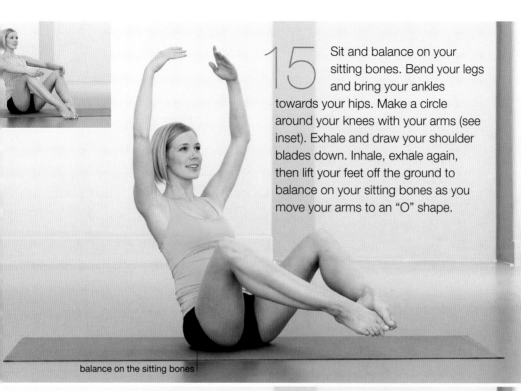

15 Sit and balance on your sitting bones. Bend your legs and bring your ankles towards your hips. Make a circle around your knees with your arms (see inset). Exhale and draw your shoulder blades down. Inhale, exhale again, then lift your feet off the ground to balance on your sitting bones as you move your arms to an "O" shape.

balance on the sitting bones

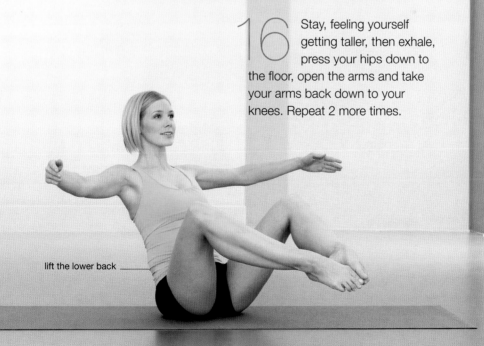

16 Stay, feeling yourself getting taller, then exhale, press your hips down to the floor, open the arms and take your arms back down to your knees. Repeat 2 more times.

lift the lower back

>> **prone rocker**

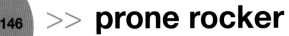

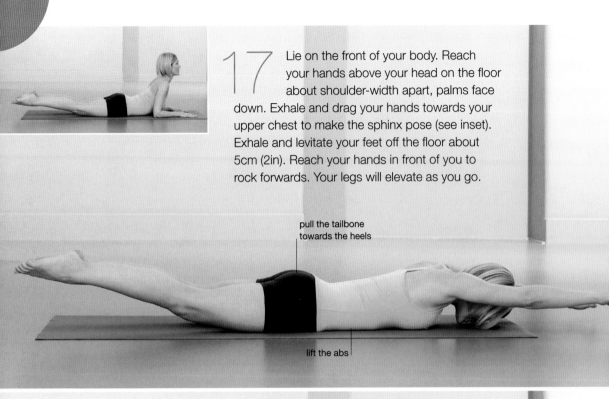

17 Lie on the front of your body. Reach your hands above your head on the floor about shoulder-width apart, palms face down. Exhale and drag your hands towards your upper chest to make the sphinx pose (see inset). Exhale and levitate your feet off the floor about 5cm (2in). Reach your hands in front of you to rock forwards. Your legs will elevate as you go.

pull the tailbone towards the heels

lift the abs

18 Lift up your head and push back up to catch yourself on your hands. Your legs will descend. Rock forwards and back for 5 more repetitions. Hold the last position to stabilize your body, then relax.

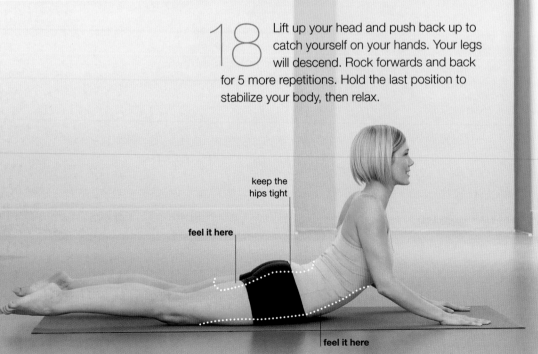

keep the hips tight

feel it here

feel it here

>> **revitalizing the back**

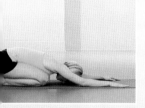

19 Kneel on the floor and bend forwards, stretching your arms along the floor above your head (see inset). Push back, allow your knees to open a little, then bring your hips back towards your heels. Place your palms one on top of the other underneath your forehead.

bring the hips towards the heels —

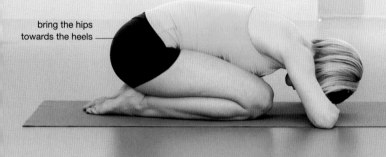

20 Inhale, push down on your hands, curl your head and round your back under, breathing in for 3 counts. Allow your hips to lift away from your feet a little. Bow your head and look towards your navel. Then exhale and lower your head and hips back towards the floor. Take 3 more in- and out-breaths as you perform this lifting and lowering motion.

let the hips lift —

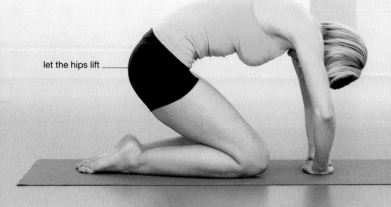

>> plank balance

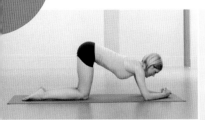

21 Go onto your forearms and knees, holding your hands together (see inset). Feel imaginary hands sandwiching your lower back. Exhale and reach your right foot behind you until your knee is straight, then reach your left foot behind you. Tuck your toes under to form 2 little stands. This is a forearm plank.

take the tailbone towards the heels

don't let the back curve

lift out of the shoulders

22 Exhale and balance on your left leg, pointing your toes of your right foot to the wall behind you. Breathe, then bring your right toes back under to the forearm plank position. Repeat to the other side, balancing on your right leg, then repeat to both sides once more.

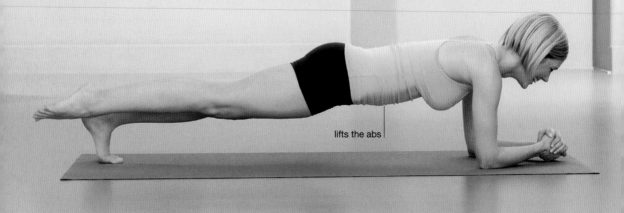

lifts the abs

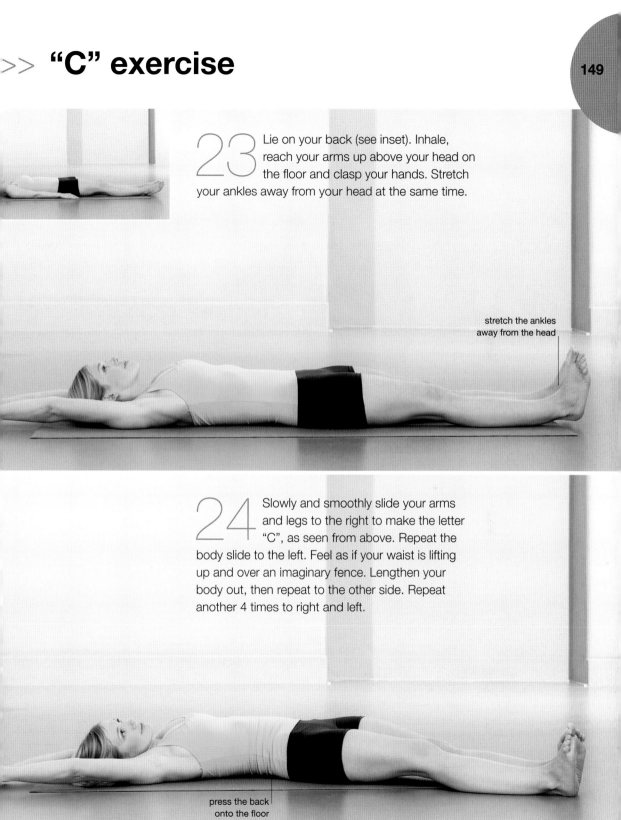

23 Lie on your back (see inset). Inhale, reach your arms up above your head on the floor and clasp your hands. Stretch your ankles away from your head at the same time.

stretch the ankles away from the head

24 Slowly and smoothly slide your arms and legs to the right to make the letter "C", as seen from above. Repeat the body slide to the left. Feel as if your waist is lifting up and over an imaginary fence. Lengthen your body out, then repeat to the other side. Repeat another 4 times to right and left.

press the back onto the floor

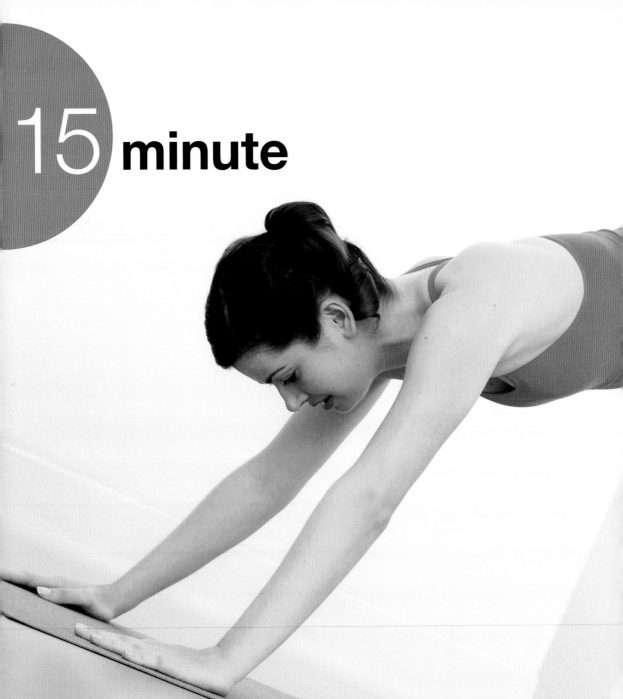

15 minute

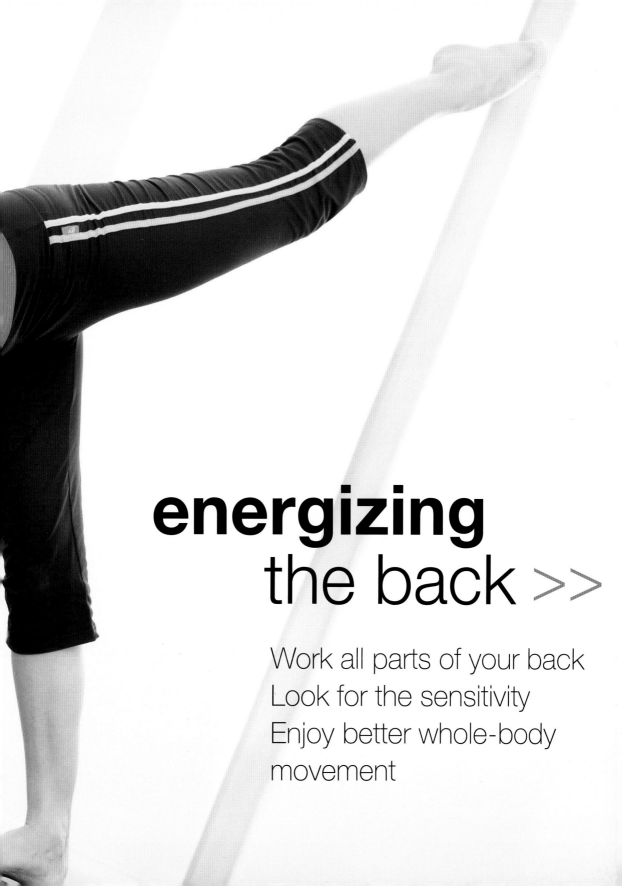

energizing
the back >>

Work all parts of your back
Look for the sensitivity
Enjoy better whole-body
movement

>> arm circles

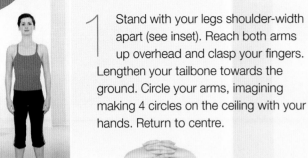

1 Stand with your legs shoulder-width apart (see inset). Reach both arms up overhead and clasp your fingers. Lengthen your tailbone towards the ground. Circle your arms, imagining making 4 circles on the ceiling with your hands. Return to centre.

2 Again, lift up and out of your waist and tighten your waist. Lengthen your tailbone. Reverse the movement with your hands, imagining making 4 more circles on the ceiling. Bring your arms down.

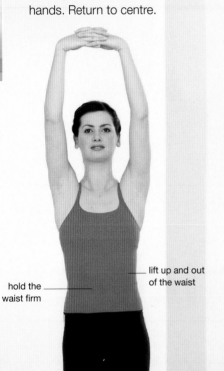

hold the waist firm

lift up and out of the waist

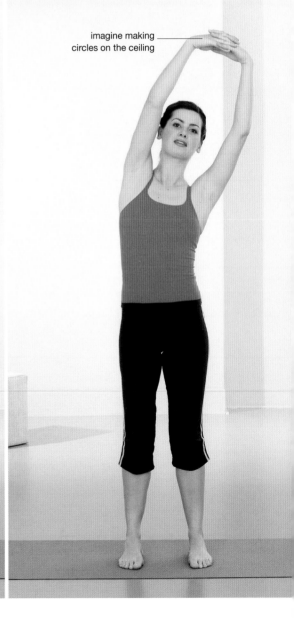

imagine making circles on the ceiling

3 Stand with your legs about shoulder-width apart (see inset). Place your hands on your hips. Start moving your hips in a circling motion. Notice that your knees will also circle at the same time. Keep them a little bent. Be sure to tighten your waist. Circle your hips one way 5 times.

4 Still keeping your knees bent and your waist tight, circle your hips the other way 5 times. Repeat the hip circles again 5 times in each direction.

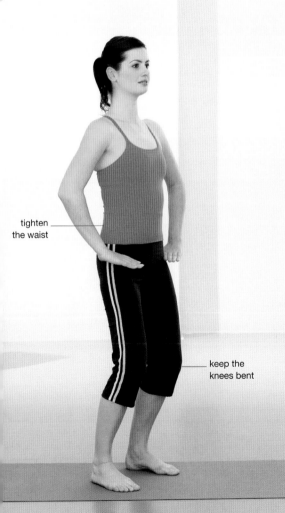

tighten the waist

keep the knees bent

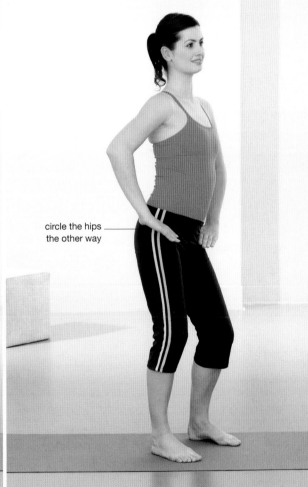

circle the hips the other way

>> **wrist and ankle circles**

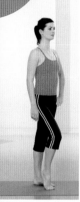

5 Stand with your legs about shoulder-width apart. Place your left hand on your left hip joint (see inset). Slowly shift onto your left leg, raise your right and find your balance. Tighten in your waist to help with the balance or hold onto a chair. Press your left foot into the ground.

6 Circle the right ankle and right wrist at the same time. Circle 5 times. Reverse the direction for 5 circles. Repeat the whole exercise again, then shift onto the right leg and repeat, circling with the left foot and left hand. Take your left leg down to the floor.

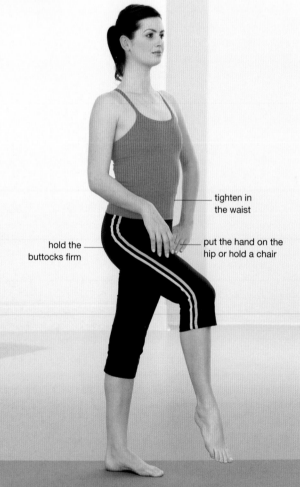

tighten in the waist

hold the buttocks firm

put the hand on the hip or hold a chair

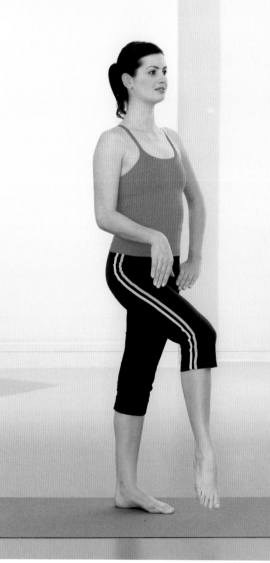

back stretch

7 Stand tall with your feet just less than hip-width apart (see inset). Take your head over your pelvis. Pull your navel inward toward your spine. Make fists with your hands and place your knuckles on your lower back. Exhale a little, then inhale as you lift your chest diagonally towards the ceiling.

8 Breathe, then return your chest and focus to look forwards again by lifting through your ears. Repeat the exercise 3 more times, inhaling as you focus up towards the ceiling and exhaling as you lengthen your spine and lift through your ears to return to look forwards. As you lift your chest, feel as if a hook is pulling your breastbone up to the ceiling.

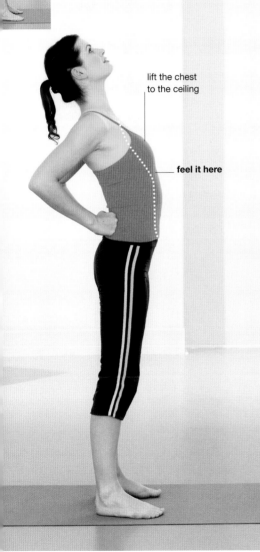

lift the chest
to the ceiling

feel it here

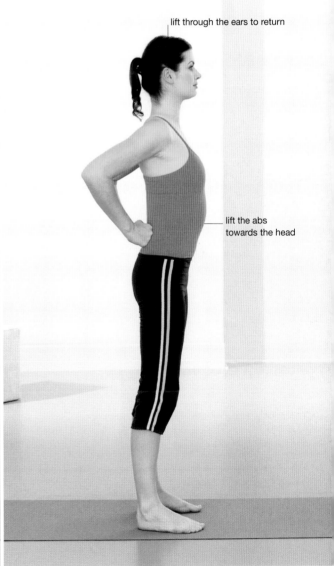

lift through the ears to return

lift the abs
towards the head

>> side stretch 3

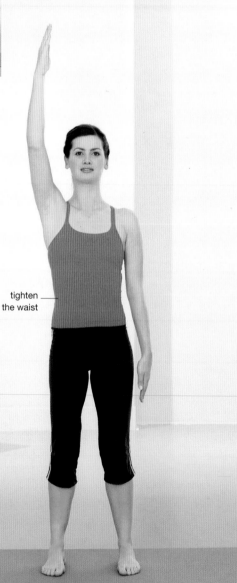

9 Stand with your feet hip-width apart (see inset). Pull your navel into your spine, drop your tailbone and bend your knees slightly. Raise your right arm and pull your right middle finger to the ceiling.

tighten the waist

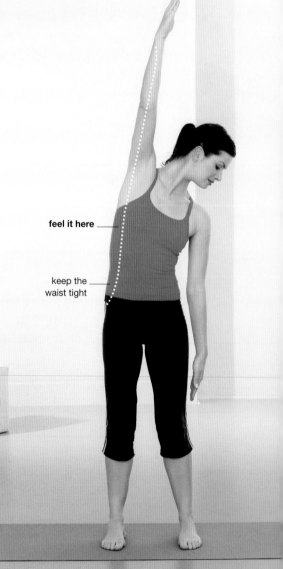

10 Look down to the left and lean and pull your left middle finger towards the floor as you reach up with your right middle finger. Elongate the whole right side of your body. Tighten and lift the pelvic floor. muscles. Take 2 breaths and then return to centre. Repeat on the other side. Return to centre again.

feel it here

keep the waist tight

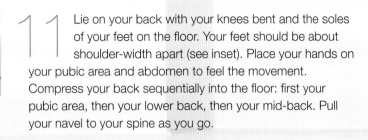

11 Lie on your back with your knees bent and the soles of your feet on the floor. Your feet should be about shoulder-width apart (see inset). Place your hands on your pubic area and abdomen to feel the movement. Compress your back sequentially into the floor: first your pubic area, then your lower back, then your mid-back. Pull your navel to your spine as you go.

hollow the pubic area

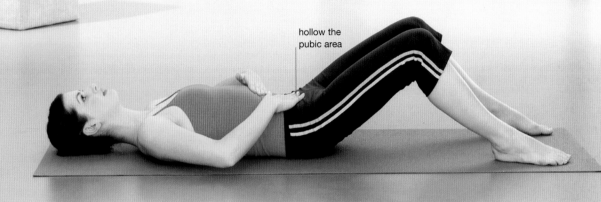

12 Imagine you are pressing pearls into sand with your back as you perform the exercise. End with a chin tuck. Hold for 4 counts, then repeat. Stretch your legs out onto the floor and take your arms behind your head. Repeat the compressions 4 times. Relax.

tuck the chin

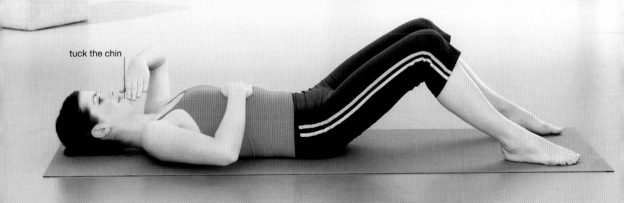

>> **puppy dog abs**

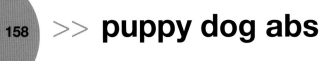

13 Lie on your back with your knees bent and arms by your sides (see inset). Hold your abs firm and lift your legs up so your shins are parallel to the floor. Bend your elbows, take your upper arms off the floor and face your palms upwards. This puppy dog position makes your core muscles work.

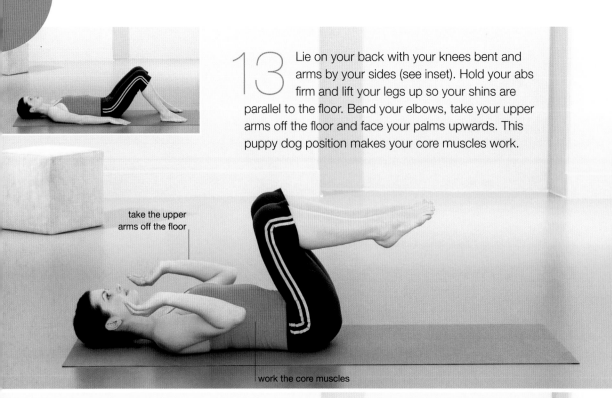

take the upper arms off the floor

work the core muscles

14 Exhale, tilt your chin, lift your head, look to your groin and lengthen your arms out past your hips. At the same time, reach your feet upwards into a "V" shape, just past shoulder-width apart. Inhale and exhale, then lower back down to the puppy dog position. Repeat the exercise 3 more times.

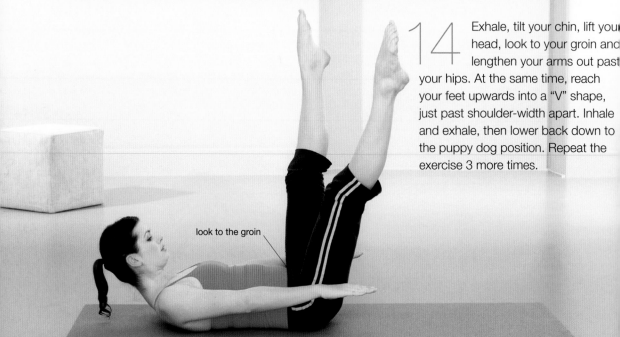

look to the groin

first position abs

15 Lie on your back in first position parallel, with your second toe in line with your kneecaps and with the midpoint on your groin line (see p120). Flex your feet. Brace with your hands at your hip joint (see inset). Lift your head to check that you are in line. Keep your head up to start the exercise.

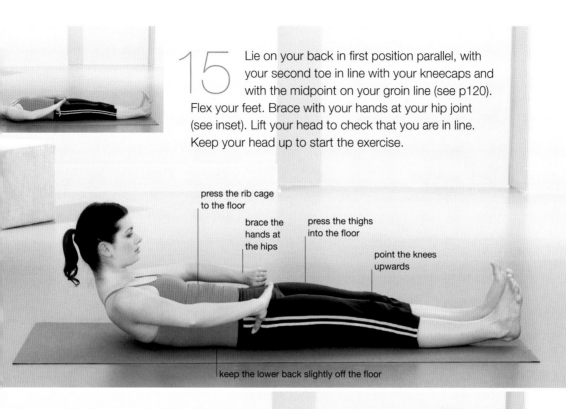

press the rib cage to the floor

brace the hands at the hips

press the thighs into the floor

point the knees upwards

keep the lower back slightly off the floor

16 Exhale as you lower your head while dragging your legs to meet at the midline of your body. Firmly press your hips, knees and ankles together, counting to 8. Repeat the lifting of your head with the opening of your legs, and the lowering of your head with pressing your legs together 3 more times. Finally, lift your head and open your legs. Relax down.

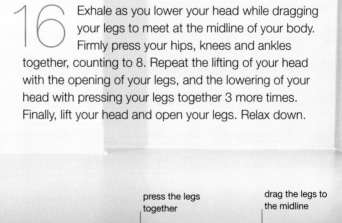

lower the head

press the legs together

drag the legs to the midline

>> hip lift

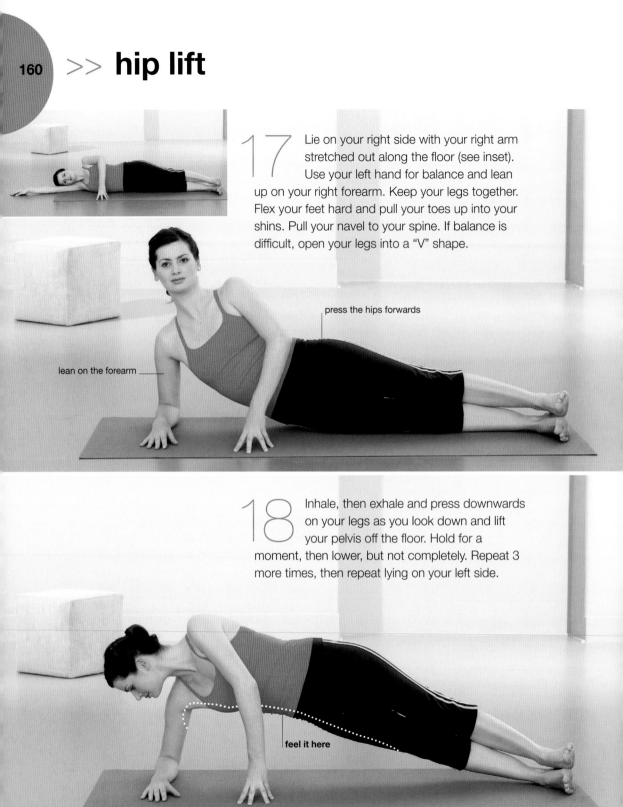

17 Lie on your right side with your right arm stretched out along the floor (see inset). Use your left hand for balance and lean up on your right forearm. Keep your legs together. Flex your feet hard and pull your toes up into your shins. Pull your navel to your spine. If balance is difficult, open your legs into a "V" shape.

press the hips forwards

lean on the forearm

18 Inhale, then exhale and press downwards on your legs as you look down and lift your pelvis off the floor. Hold for a moment, then lower, but not completely. Repeat 3 more times, then repeat lying on your left side.

feel it here

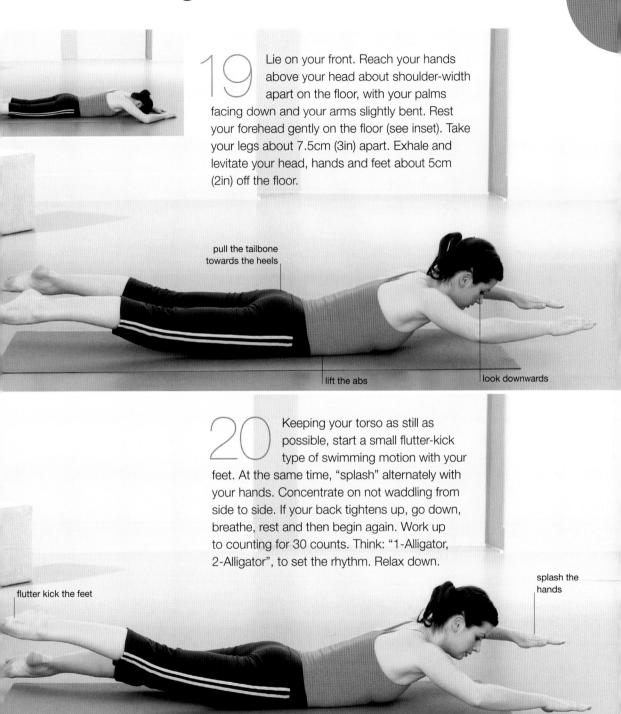

19 Lie on your front. Reach your hands above your head about shoulder-width apart on the floor, with your palms facing down and your arms slightly bent. Rest your forehead gently on the floor (see inset). Take your legs about 7.5cm (3in) apart. Exhale and levitate your head, hands and feet about 5cm (2in) off the floor.

pull the tailbone towards the heels

lift the abs

look downwards

20 Keeping your torso as still as possible, start a small flutter-kick type of swimming motion with your feet. At the same time, "splash" alternately with your hands. Concentrate on not waddling from side to side. If your back tightens up, go down, breathe, rest and then begin again. Work up to counting for 30 counts. Think: "1-Alligator, 2-Alligator", to set the rhythm. Relax down.

splash the hands

flutter kick the feet

>> inverted stretch

21 Go onto all fours, then tuck you toes under and lift your knees off the floor to come up into ar upside-down triangle. Touching your toes of your right foot to the floor (see inset), ex transfer almost all your weight into your rig hand, and raise your right leg up behind yo

keep the right hip low

22 Slowly open your right leg to y right side while keeping weigh the right hand. Press into you right hand as you return the foot behind yo Give your foot a little lift, lengthen, then lov Repeat with your left leg.

keep the leg parallel to the floor

>> hanging stretch

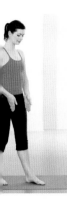

23 Stand with your legs about 7.5cm (3in) apart. Place your left foot ahead of your right with about a foot's width between the legs. The toes point forwards (see inset). Cross your arms, hold your elbows and pull your navel firmly into the spine. Reach the elbows downwards.

24 Continue to reach the elbows down towards the floor. Stay in this rounded position, firmly holding your abs as you take 3 breaths. Carefully roll up, feeling as if your abs are walking up the front of your body. Repeat on the other side. Come back up and relax.

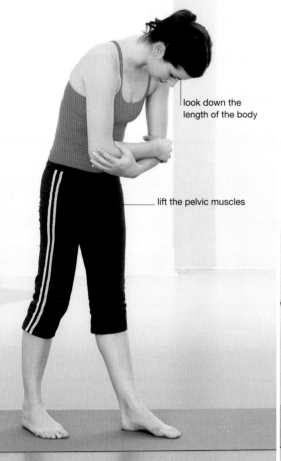

look down the length of the body

lift the pelvic muscles

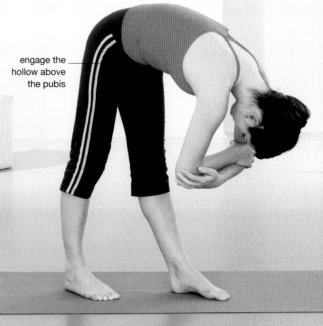

engage the hollow above the pubis

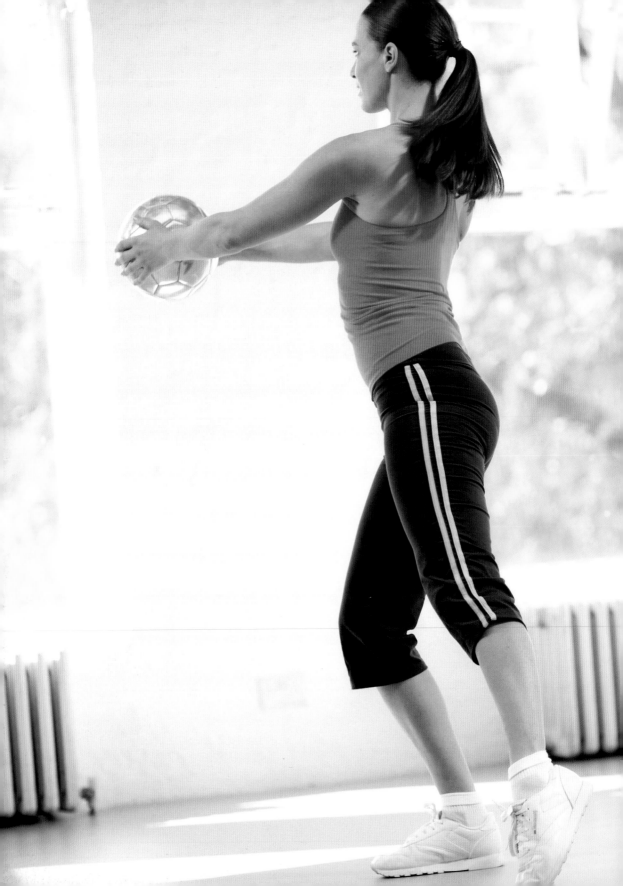

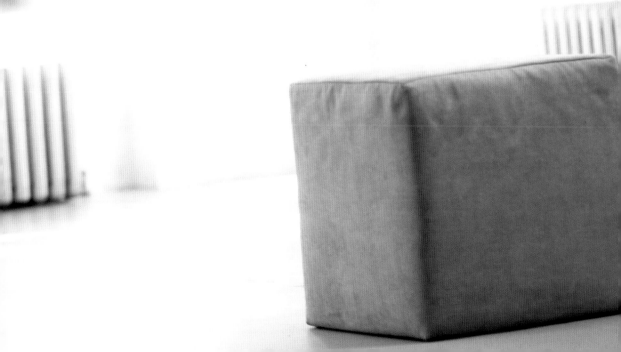

>> **15** minute

total body
workout

Joan Pagano

>> working the total body

No more excuses! It's time to get moving. Do you think you're too busy, can't afford it, or don't have enough room or equipment to work out at home? Maybe you feel it's too boring, not fun, and you can't stick with it? Or that you're too lazy, old, fat, or out of shape to even begin?

The list of excuses not to get fit is endless, but the solution is simple: *Total Body Workout* provides the tools you need for an exercise programme with minimal investment of time and resources, and from which you will definitely benefit.

15-minute workouts

The *Total Body Workout* exercise routines are designed to give you maximum benefit in the most efficient format, combining cardio and strength training. All it takes to complete a full-body routine is 15 minutes. Therefore, if 15 minutes is all you have, choose just one of them. Or, if you have more time, combine the routines for a 30-minute workout. Choose your workout according to your level of fitness, energy, and available time.

Each of the two 15-minute workouts has a unique theme to make it more enjoyable and offer variety to your routines. They challenge your body in different ways: Toning Ball (see p256) uses a ball in a variety of sporty moves. Hop, Jig, and Jump (see p272) evokes the childlike joy of jumping.

The formula for each of the workout is consistent: a three-minute warm up, followed by 10 minutes of strength (or resistance) training exercises that alternate with cardio intervals, and finally a two-minute cool down. These workout routines have been carefully selected to maximize your results by impacting all aspects of fitness.

>> SMART tips for success

Goal setting is one of the best ways to stay motivated to exercise. The SMART system states that goals should be:

- **Specific** What exactly do you want to achieve? Reduce fat, improve muscle tone, increase bone density? With clear goals, you can choose appropriate exercises.

- **Measurable** Unless your goal is measurable, you won't know if you've accomplished it. Specific goals are measurable: muscle tone can be measured by endurance exercises.

- **Action-oriented** An action plan breaking your long-term goal into weekly targets will give you the satisfaction of meeting short-term goals, and the opportunity to reassess whether your goals are reasonable.

- **Realistic** People often become disillusioned and stop exercising when they don't get their imagined results. Are your goals in sync with your body type? Do they match your personal preferences?

- **Timed** Setting a target date gives you the motivation to stick with an exercise programme, but you must allow a realistic amount of time to achieve your goal.

Composition of a workout

The warm ups are a series of movements that gradually build in intensity, giving you the flavour of the workout and preparing your body for the exercises to come. The strength-training programmes comply with fitness industry guidelines that target the major hip, thigh, leg, back, chest, shoulder, arm, and abdominal muscles. The one-minute cardio intervals carry out the theme of the workout, at a higher level of intensity to pump up your heart in between the resistance exercises.

The body of the workout is composed of standing exercises for the purpose of burning more calories and preserving bone density. Many of them are combination moves involving multiple muscle groups, such as Lunge and Row (see p265), and Squat with Knee Lift (see p264). Again, the purpose is to produce the best results for your efforts: to target the most muscle groups, burn the most calories, and improve co-ordination at the same time; training your muscles to work in patterns.

No workout is complete without a full-body stretch, and this is provided in the cool down. As opposed to more traditional stretches that isolate individual muscles, these positions target multiple muscle groups, often stretching the upper and lower body together. They provide a fluid sequence as you progress through the movements.

Integrating all these aspects of training prepares your whole body to meet the demands of your day-to-day activities more effectively (i.e. functional training). You'll really appreciate it the next time you are walking home on a wet, windy day, an open umbrella in one hand, a loaded tote bag over the opposite shoulder, with several full shopping bags in the other hand, when you want to buy a newspaper without falling over. This is the payoff of functional training.

To obtain maximum benefit and prevent injury, careful attention to form and posture is essential when exercising.

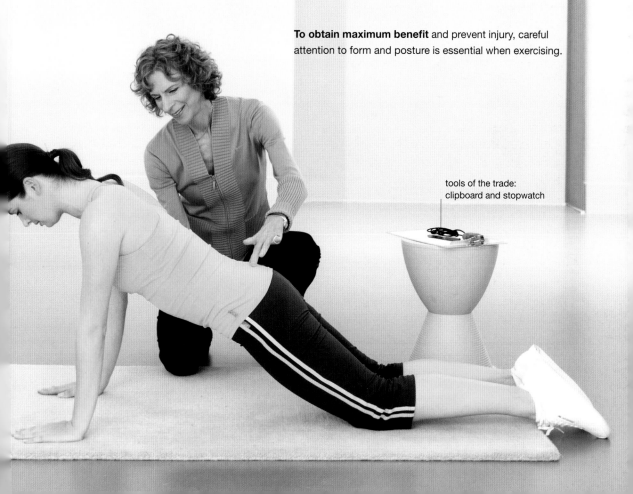

tools of the trade:
clipboard and stopwatch

>> **your training** programme

Now that you've assessed your current condition, you are ready to start making improvements to your personal level of fitness, as well as your health, appearance, energy levels, and overall mood. Each 15-minute workout combines cardio with resistance training and stretching.

Cardiovascular stamina, muscular strength and endurance, flexibility, and body composition are the aspects of physical fitness that are most closely related to health. Each of these characteristics is directly related to good health and to your risk of developing certain types of disease – notably those that are associated with inactivity.

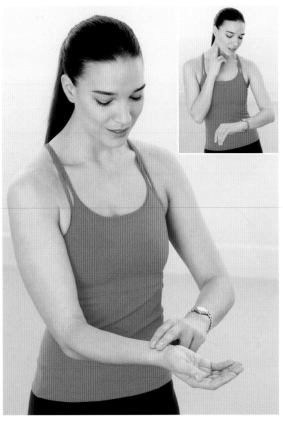

Benefits of cardiovascular fitness

A fit cardiovascular system is associated with a stronger heart muscle, slower heart rate, decreased chance of heart attack, and a greater chance of surviving if you do suffer a heart attack. Regular aerobic exercise can reduce your blood pressure and blood fats, including low-density lipids (LDL), which can help you resist build up of plaque in the arteries (atherosclerosis). It can also increase the protective high-density lipids (HDL) and improve circulation and the capacity of the blood to carry oxygen throughout your body. Improving cardiovascular fitness also decreases your risk of some cancers and of obesity, diabetes, osteoporosis, depression, and anxiety.

With training, your heart gets stronger and can pump more blood with each beat, resulting in a lower heart rate during exercise and at rest. The average resting rate is 60 to 80 beats per minute. Take your resting heart rate when you start your programme and then eight weeks later and compare the numbers. Find your pulse (see left), count the first beat as "zero" and time yourself for 30 seconds. Multiply the score by two to arrive at the number of beats per minute.

Taking your pulse To take your pulse at the wrist (the "radial pulse") place your index and middle fingers on the palm side of the opposite wrist. Alternatively, you can take your pulse at the neck (the "carotid pulse"), just below the jaw bone to the side of the larynx.

Muscle strength and endurance

Muscular strength (the ability to exert force) and endurance (the ability of the muscles to exert themselves repeatedly) allow you to work more efficiently and to resist fatigue, muscle soreness, and back problems. Strengthening the muscles and joints allows you to increase the intensity and duration of your cardiovascular training. As you work the muscles, you simultaneously stimulate the bones to build and maintain density, decreasing the risk of developing osteoporosis.

Stretching and flexibility

Your ability to stretch out the muscles and maintain range of motion in the joints is another aspect of muscular fitness. Stretching helps improve posture by correcting the tendency of certain muscles to shorten and tighten; it counteracts the physical stressors of our day-to-day activities and discharges tension from the muscles.

Frequency and duration

For resistance training you need to do a minimum of two 15-minute sessions per week, and no muscle should be worked more than three times in one week. Allow a day of rest in between working each muscle group, since the repair and recovery of the muscle fibres is as important as the stress to the development of the muscle. The length of your session will vary from 15 to 60 minutes, depending on your initial fitness and available time.

Maintenance programme

Periodically, you should vary the workouts you choose or the order you perform them in so that you keep your muscles "alert." You may also want to increase your weights, but be aware that this may trigger problems in the neck, shoulder, elbow, lower back, or knee. You may be able to cope with heavier weights in some muscle groups, but not in others, so experiment carefully. Posture and alignment, and core conditioning are also important aspects of your training.

>> myths about weight training

● **Myth 1**
Lifting weights will make you bulk up.

Truth Only if you have high levels of testosterone and use very heavy weights. Most women lack the necessary hormones and strength to build significant muscle mass.

● **Myth 2**
You shouldn't lift weights if you are an older adult, overweight, or out of shape.

Truth Not so! Weight training can help you rejuvenate, lose weight, and shape up.

● **Myth 3**
A thin person does not need to build lean body mass by lifting weights.

Truth Appearances are deceiving when it comes to body composition, and being thin is no guarantee that you are lean. Without weight training, you steadily lose muscle and gain fat as you age.

● **Myth 4**
Certain weight-training exercises can help you spot reduce.

Truth You can spot strengthen and shape a body area, but fat belongs to the whole body and needs to be reduced all over, through expending more calories (aerobic exercise and weight training) than you consume.

● **Myth 5**
Aerobic activities, not weight training, are the most efficient type of exercise to lose weight.

Truth Losing weight requires a balanced exercise programme of aerobic exercise to burn calories and weight training to speed up the metabolism.

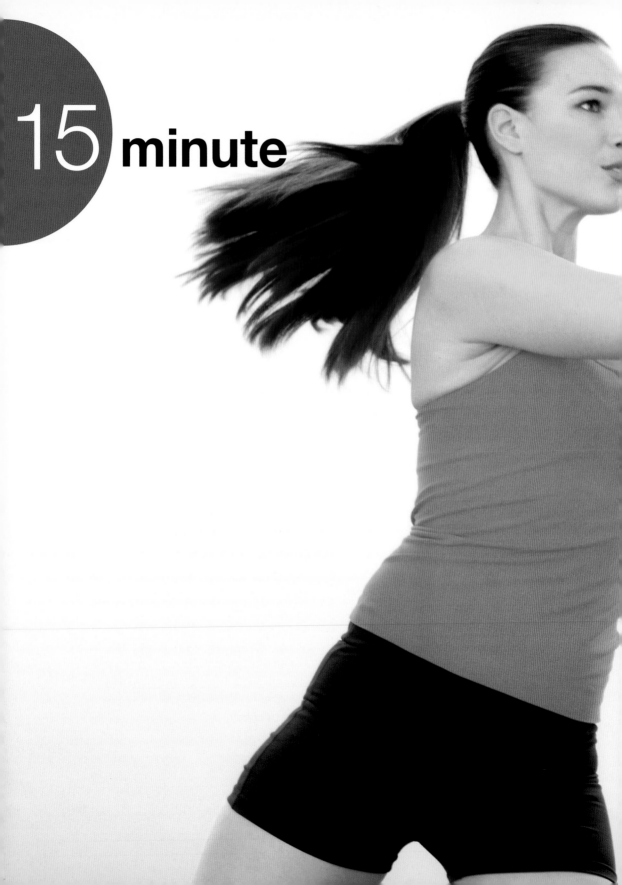

15 minute

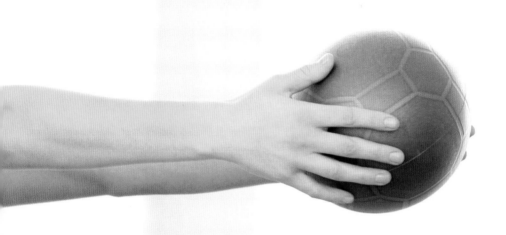

toning ball
workout >>

Improve your coordination
and balance
Add variety to your workout
with a ball

>> rock lunge/skater

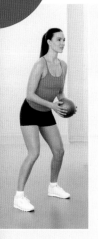

1 To begin your warm up, stand with your feet parallel, slightly wider than shoulder width apart, knees bent. Lean forwards slightly and hold the ball in front of your hips (see inset). Straighten one leg and lunge the other way, moving the ball to your opposite hip. Repeat, alternating sides for a total of 8 reps (1 rep = both sides).

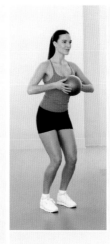

2 Stand with your feet parallel, hip-width apart, knees bent. Hold the ball in front of your chest (see inset). Keep one knee bent and shift your weight onto it as you extend the other leg out to the side, toe resting lightly on the floor. Stretch your arms out diagonally, pressing the ball away from your extended leg. Then return to the starting position and repeat, alternating sides, for a total of 8 reps (1 rep = both sides).

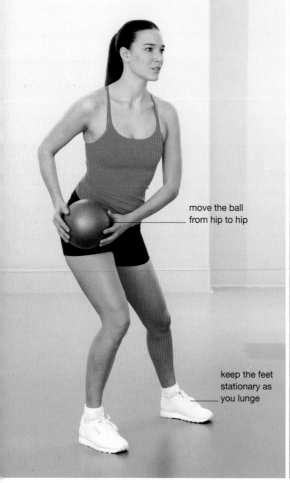

move the ball from hip to hip

keep the feet stationary as you lunge

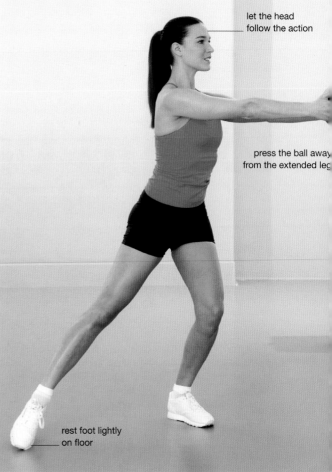

let the head follow the action

press the ball away from the extended leg

rest foot lightly on floor

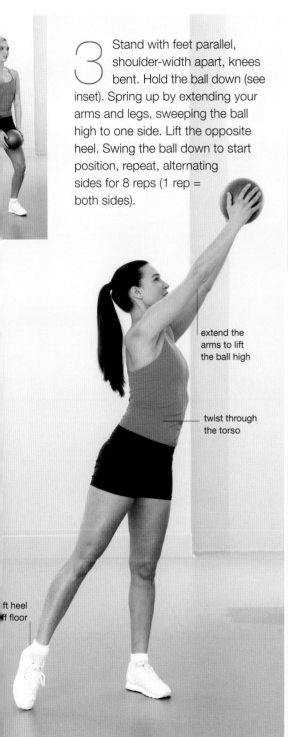

3 Stand with feet parallel, shoulder-width apart, knees bent. Hold the ball down (see inset). Spring up by extending your arms and legs, sweeping the ball high to one side. Lift the opposite heel. Swing the ball down to start position, repeat, alternating sides for 8 reps (1 rep = both sides).

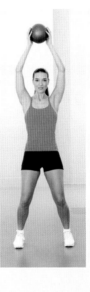

4 Stand with feet parallel, shoulder-width apart, knees slightly bent. Hold the ball overhead (see inset). Step one leg inwards and flex at the waist, swinging the ball to the same side. Repeat, alternating sides, for a total of 8 reps (1 rep = both sides).

extend the arms to lift the ball high

twist through the torso

ft heel f floor

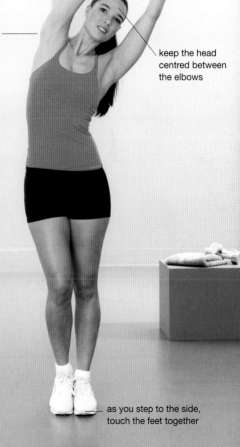

draw the shoulder blades down

keep the head centred between the elbows

as you step to the side, touch the feet together

>> wood-chop squat/curl and press

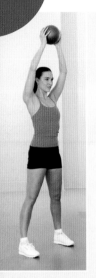

5 Still holding the ball above your head, stand with your feet parallel, shoulder-width apart, knees soft (see inset). Bend your knees into a squat, reaching back with your hips, keeping your heels pressed into the floor. With your arms straight, "chop" the ball down, lowering it to the knees. Repeat 8 times.

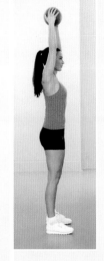

6 Reach the ball towards the ceiling (see inset), then bend both elbows, lowering it behind your head. At the same time, bend one leg back, lifting your heel towards the buttocks. Repeat, alternating legs, for a total of 8 reps (1 rep = both sides). **Repeat Steps 5–1** (reverse order) to complete your warm up.

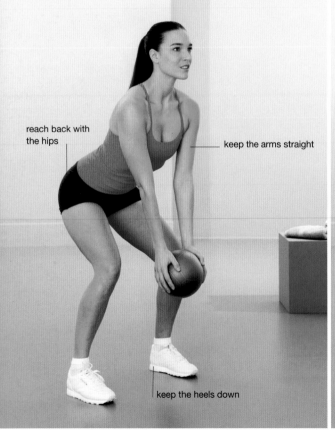

reach back with the hips

keep the arms straight

keep the heels down

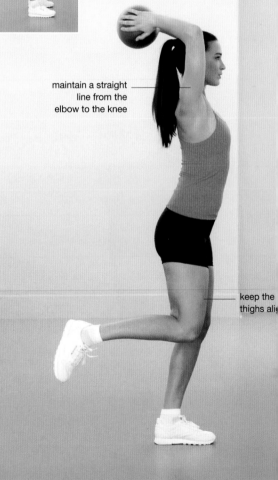

maintain a straight line from the elbow to the knee

keep the thighs ali[g]

>> plié with front raise

7a Put down the ball and pick up one large weight for the first resistance exercise. Stand with your feet slightly wider than shoulder-width apart, shift your weight to your heels, and turn your legs out from the hips until your feet are at 45-degree angles. Hold the weight horizontally with one hand at each end, your arms straight down in front.

7b As you inhale, bend your knees until your thighs are as parallel to the floor as possible; simultaneously lift the weight to shoulder height, keeping your arms straight. Exhale, press through your heels, and tighten your inner and outer thighs as you return to the starting position. Repeat 12 times.

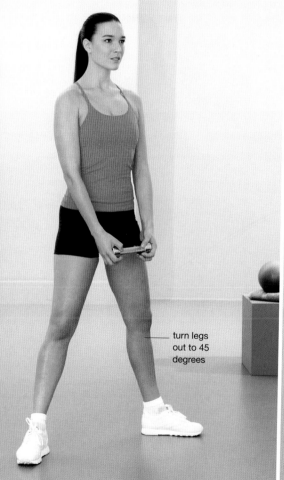

turn legs out to 45 degrees

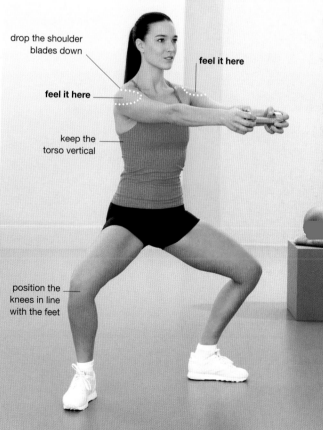

drop the shoulder blades down

feel it here

feel it here

keep the torso vertical

position the knees in line with the feet

>> **step and dig/knee lift**

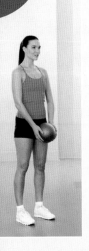

8 Start your first cardio interval. Stand with your feet hip-width apart, knees soft, feet parallel or slightly turned out. Hold the ball with your arms straight down (see inset). Tap your heel to the front, pointing your toes to the ceiling, as you bring the ball up to shoulder height. Keep your arms straight, not stiff. Alternate legs for a total of 8 reps (1 rep = both sides). Breathe naturally.

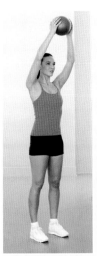

9 Stand with your feet parallel, hip-width apart, knees slightly bent. Hold the ball above your head, with elbows slightly rounded (see inset). Bring your knee up to hip height as you lower the ball towards your knee. Repeat, alternating legs for 8 reps (1 rep = both sides). Breathe naturally throughout.

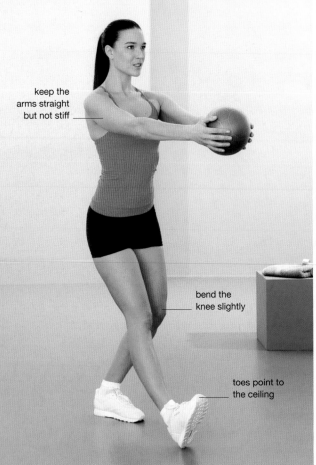

keep the arms straight but not stiff

bend the knee slightly

toes point to the ceiling

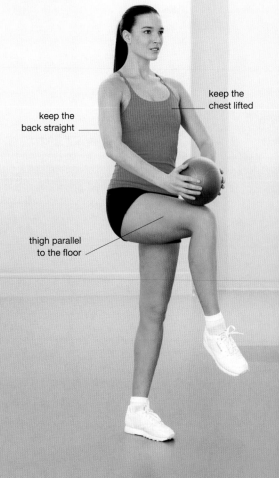

keep the chest lifted

keep the back straight

thigh parallel to the floor

>> **squat plus**

10a Stand with your feet shoulder-width apart, holding the ball with your arms straight down (see inset). Bend your knees into a squat, at the same time bending your elbows to lift the ball to your chest. Keep your weight centred, heels down. Reach back with your hips, keeping your knees behind your toes.

10b Lift the ball up above your head as you straighten your legs (see inset). Then bend into the squat, ball to chest (see 10a), before returning to the starting position. Take full, deep breaths. Repeat the sequence 12 times. **Steps 8–10 complete the cardio interval.**

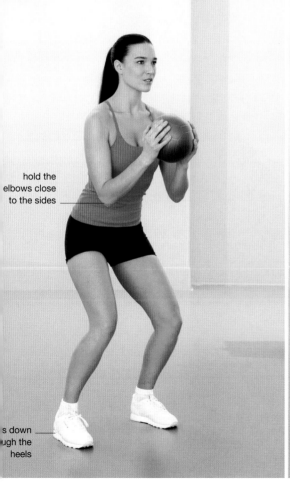

hold the
elbows close
to the sides

s down
ugh the
heels

keep the
shoulders down

keep the
back straight

straighten the legs

>> squat with knee lift

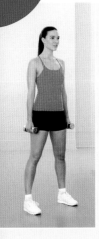

11a Put down the beach ball and pick up two large free weights. Stand with your feet parallel, shoulder-width apart, knees soft. Hold one weight in each hand, with your arms by your sides and palms facing in (see inset). Inhale as you squat: shift your weight back into your heels, reaching back with your hips and letting your torso lean forwards. Release your pelvis to allow a natural curve in your back.

11b Exhale and straighten your legs. Shift your weight to one side and bring the other knee up to hip height. Balance for a moment, then return to the starting position (see inset, left). Squat again (see left), straighten your legs, and change sides for the knee lift (see below). Keep your hips level, chest lifted, eyes forwards throughout. Repeat for a total of 8 reps (1 rep = both sides). **Do your next cardio interval, steps 8–10 (pp176–177).**

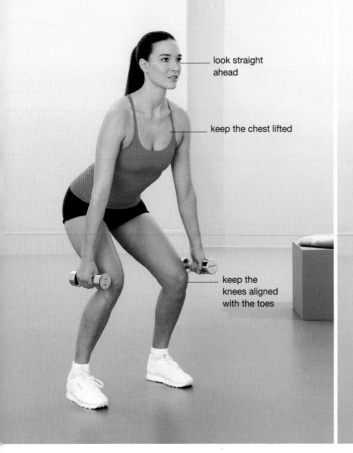

look straight ahead

keep the chest lifted

keep the knees aligned with the toes

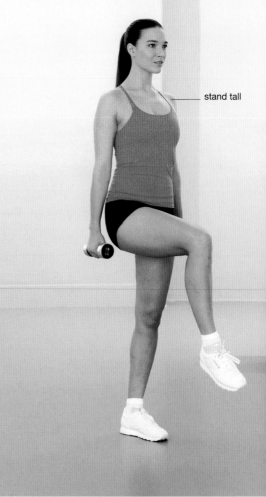

stand tall

12a Exchange the ball for two large free weights. Stand with your feet parallel, hip-width apart, knees soft. Hold the weights at your hips, palms in, elbows bent at right angles and close to your sides. Stabilize your shoulder blades by drawing them down and together. Keep your wrists straight, in line with your forearms.

12b Inhale as you step forwards with one leg, bending both knees. At the same time, straighten your arms, lowering the weights towards your knee. Exhale as you spring back, pulling the weights to your hips. Alternate legs for 8 reps (1 rep = both sides). **Do the next cardio interval, steps 8–10 (pp176–177).**

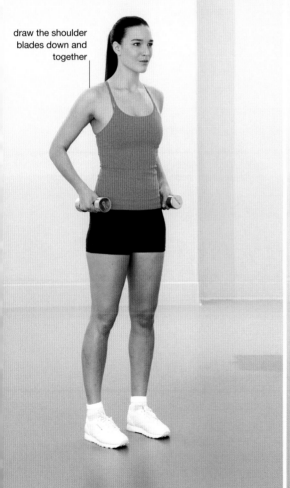

draw the shoulder blades down and together

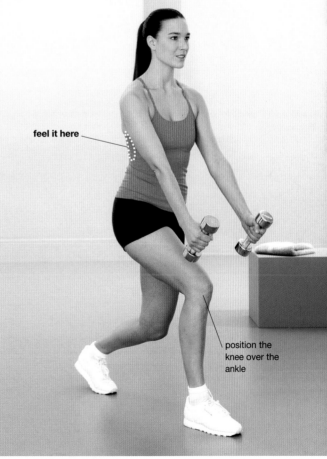

feel it here

position the knee over the ankle

>> squat with weight shift

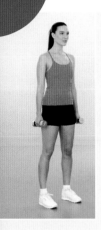

13a

Pick up two large weights. Stand with your feet parallel, hip width apart. Hold the weights by your sides. Shifting your weight into your heels, inhale as you bend your knees into a squat; at the same time, bend your elbows, bringing the weights up towards your shoulders.

13b

Exhale as you straighten your arms and legs to the starting position. Inhale again, then exhale as you shift your weight onto the balls of your feet and lift your heels high. Balance for a moment before lowering the heels onto the floor and preparing for the next squat. Do 8 reps, combining both moves. **Then do your next cardio interval, steps 8–10 (pp176–177).**

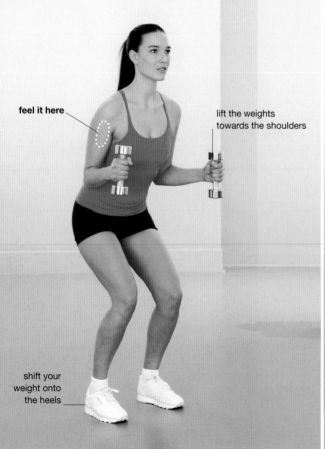

feel it here

lift the weights towards the shoulders

shift your weight onto the heels

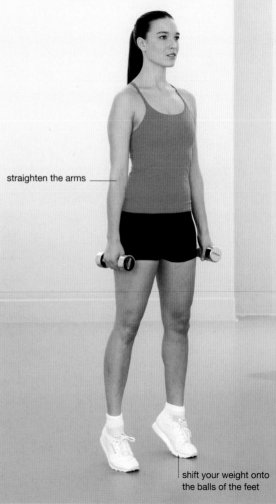

straighten the arms

shift your weight onto the balls of the feet

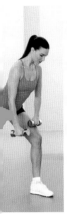

14 Exchange the ball for two large free weights. Stand in staggered lunge position, one foot forwards and the arm on the same side resting on your thigh (see inset). Draw your shoulder blade in and exhale as you lift the other arm out to the side at shoulder height. Repeat 12 times, then switch sides. **Do your next cardio interval, steps 8–10 (pp176–177).**

15 Exchange the ball for two large weights. Bend your knees and hinge forwards. Bend your elbows to 90 degrees and raise your upper arms parallel to the floor (see inset). Exhale, extending forearms behind. Inhale as you bend your elbows. Repeat 12 times. **Do your next cardio interval, Steps 8–10 (pp176–177).**

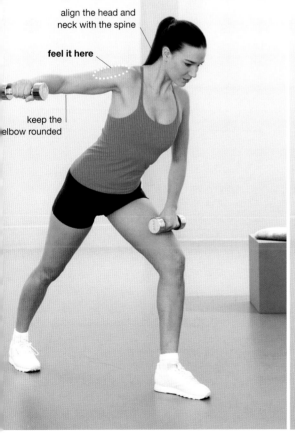

align the head and neck with the spine

feel it here

keep the elbow rounded

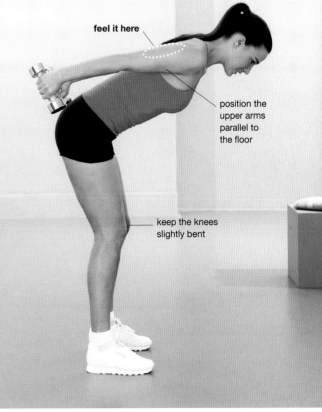

feel it here

position the upper arms parallel to the floor

keep the knees slightly bent

>> lat stretch/triceps stretch

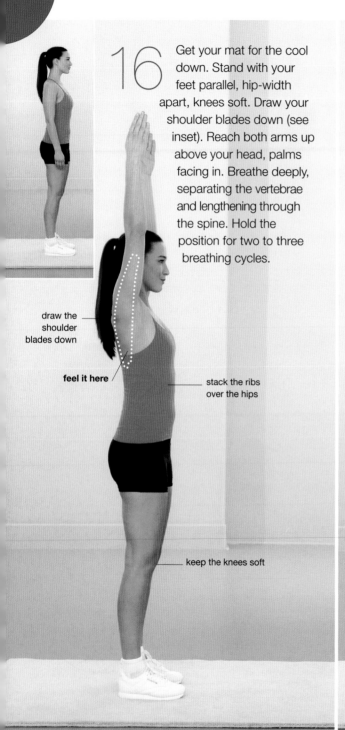

16 Get your mat for the cool down. Stand with your feet parallel, hip-width apart, knees soft. Draw your shoulder blades down (see inset). Reach both arms up above your head, palms facing in. Breathe deeply, separating the vertebrae and lengthening through the spine. Hold the position for two to three breathing cycles.

draw the shoulder blades down

feel it here

stack the ribs over the hips

keep the knees soft

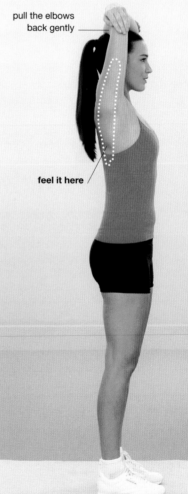

17 Cross your arms and take hold of your elbows. Keep your head centred. Gently pull your elbows back and hold. If this is too difficult, hold one elbow at a time. Use a steady stretch without bouncing to allow the muscle to lengthen gradually. Breathe deeply.

pull the elbows back gently

feel it here

18 Still holding your elbows, and with your head centred, lift up from the waist and bend to one side, feeling a stretch all the way down your side to the hip. Hold, breathing into the stretch; then pass through the centre and bend to the other side. Hold, take a deep breath and then return to centre.

19 From the centre position reach forward with your arms at shoulder height. Cross your wrists and turn your palms inwards to bring them together, thumbs facing down. Round your upper back, head and neck aligned with your spine, ears between your upper arms. Separate your shoulder blades and reach as far forward as possible. Breathe and relax deeper into the stretch with each exhalation.

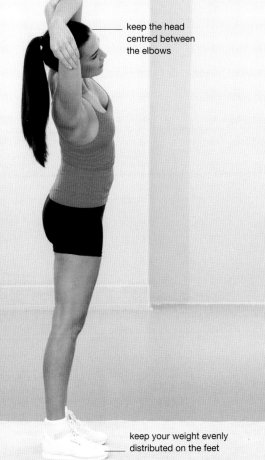

keep the head centred between the elbows

keep your weight evenly distributed on the feet

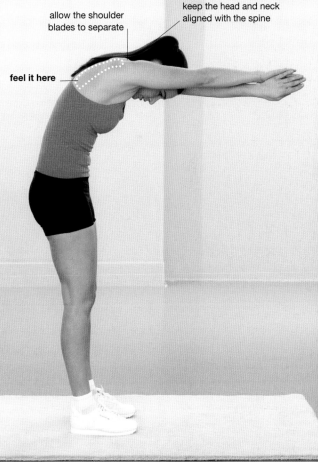

allow the shoulder blades to separate

keep the head and neck aligned with the spine

feel it here

>> spinal roll-down/downward dog

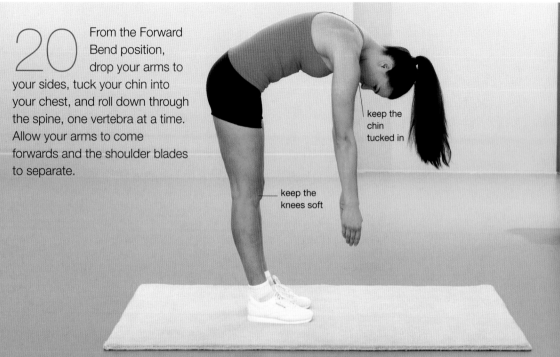

20 From the Forward Bend position, drop your arms to your sides, tuck your chin into your chest, and roll down through the spine, one vertebra at a time. Allow your arms to come forwards and the shoulder blades to separate.

keep the chin tucked in

keep the knees soft

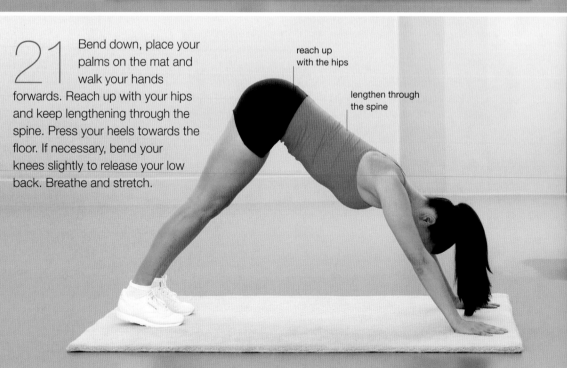

21 Bend down, place your palms on the mat and walk your hands forwards. Reach up with your hips and keep lengthening through the spine. Press your heels towards the floor. If necessary, bend your knees slightly to release your low back. Breathe and stretch.

reach up with the hips

lengthen through the spine

22 Walk forwards and place your forearms on the mat, elbows directly under your shoulders, palms facing in, hands in loose fists. Tighten your abdominal and back muscles to keep your torso lifted in a straight line from head to toe. Tuck your toes under slightly: you will feel a stretch in your calves. Hold the position, breathing naturally.

keep the shoulder blades down

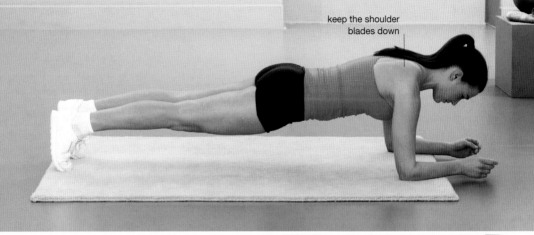

23 Bend your knees and reach back with your hips until your buttocks rest on your heels. At the same time round forwards, curving the spine, forehead towards floor. Reach your arms to the front to stretch your lats, chest, and shoulders. With every exhale, sink deeper into the position; mind and body calm. Move back into the plank, bending your elbows and straightening your legs. Finally, repeat the Child's Pose to complete your cool down.

feel it here

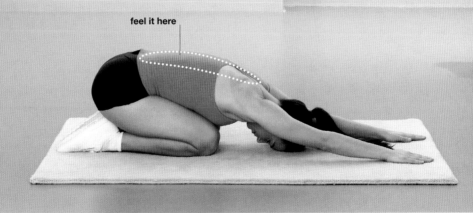

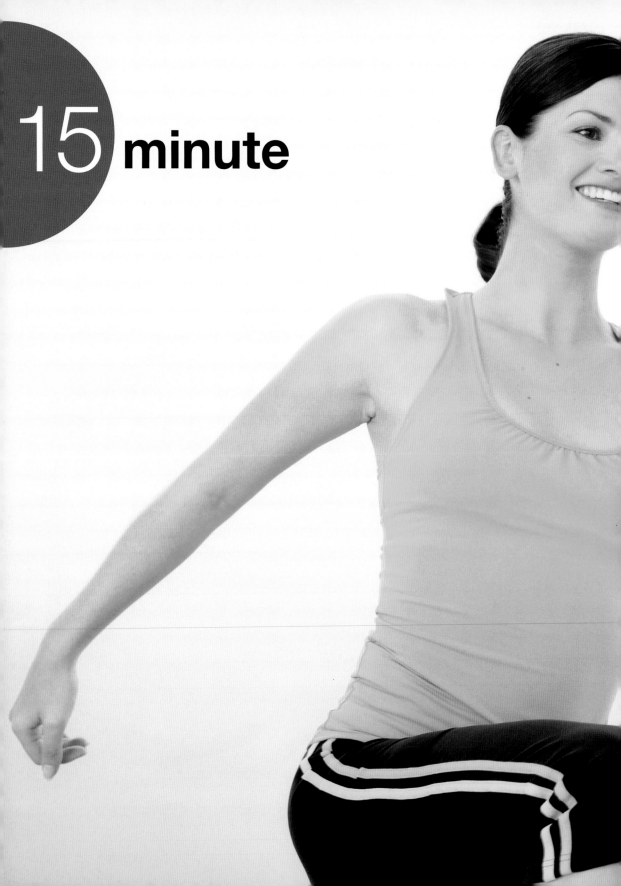

15 minute

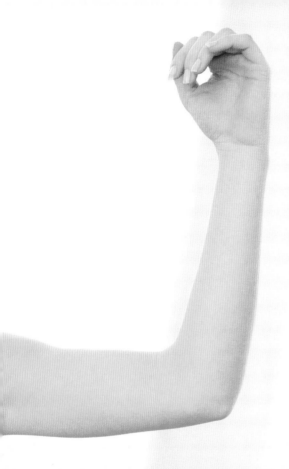

hop, jig, & jump
workout >>

Experience the childlike joy
of hopping and jumping
Release endorphins with this
upbeat workout

>> bend and raise/double arm swing

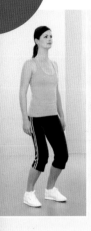

1 To warm up, stand with your feet parallel, hip-width apart, knees soft, arms by your sides. Tighten your abs and lift your chest. Bend your knees (see inset) then straighten your legs. Shift your weight to the balls of your feet and lift your heels, resisting the floor. Continue bending and then rising up, allowing your arms to swing naturally forwards, for a total of 8 times.

2 Continue to bend your knees rhythmically as you swing your arms to back and front. From the starting position of bent knees (see inset, left), feet flat on the floor, straighten your legs and swing your arms behind. Bend your knees again as your arms pass through the centre and then swing them in front as you straighten your legs. Repeat for a total of 8 swings, back to front.

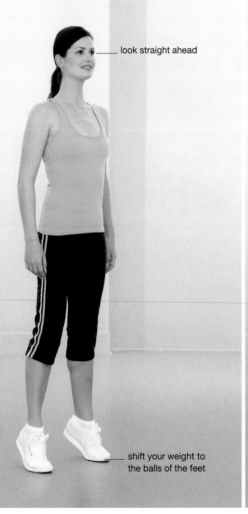

look straight ahead

shift your weight to the balls of the feet

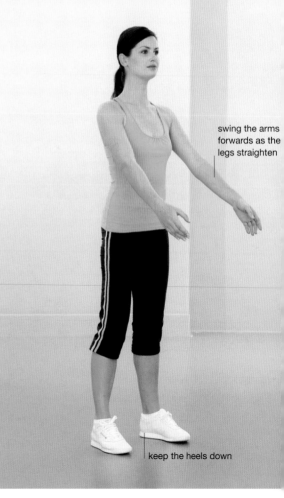

swing the arms forwards as the legs straighten

keep the heels down

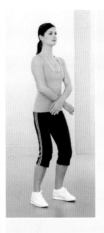

3 Continue to bend your knees rhythmically (see inset), but change the arms, swinging one forwards and the other back every time you straighten your legs. Keep your heels down, knees in line with toes. Keep your shoulder blades down as you swing your arms. Your chest stays lifted, chin level. Repeat, alternating arms, for a total of 8 reps (1 rep = both sides).

4 Continuing with rhythmic knee bends, change your arms to cross in front as you bend your knees (see inset) and then lift them out to the sides as you straighten your legs. Keep your shoulder blades down as you lift your arms to shoulder height, palms down. Bend and straighten, lifting your arms out to the sides, 16 times.

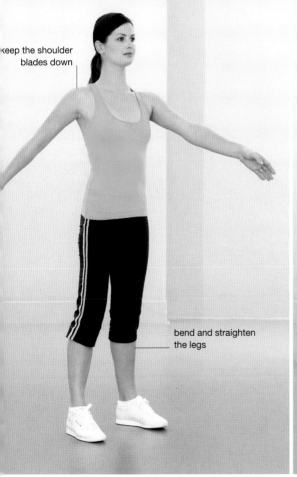

keep the shoulder blades down

bend and straighten the legs

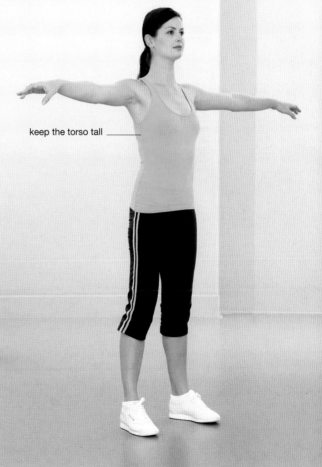

keep the torso tall

>> lateral lift/jumping jack

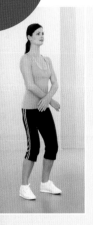

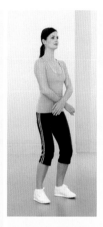

5 Arms stay the same as you bend and straighten your knees, but you add a side leg lift. Bend your knees as you cross your arms in front (see inset), then straighten both legs and lift one to the side as you raise your arms. Keep your hips level, shoulders down. Repeat, alternating legs, for a total of 8 reps (1 rep = both sides).

6 Continue to raise and lower your arms, but change your legs. As you cross your arms in front (see inset), jump your feet together. As you raise your arms to shoulder height, tap one foot out to the side. Alternate sides for 8 reps (1 rep = both sides). **Repeat steps 5–1** (reverse order) to complete your warm up.

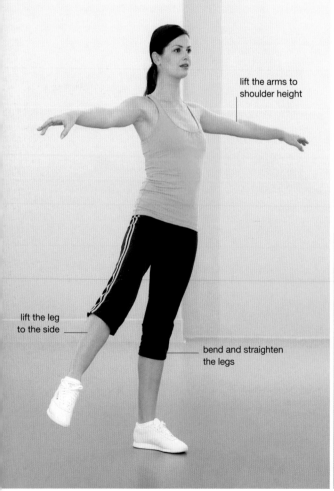

lift the arms to shoulder height

lift the leg to the side

bend and straighten the legs

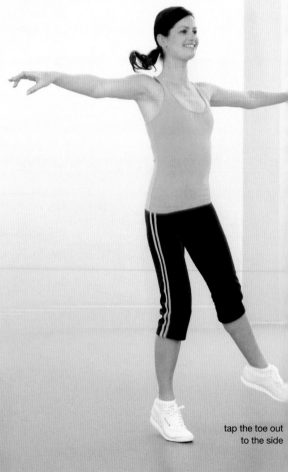

tap the toe out to the side

7a Pick up two small weights for your first resistance exercise. Stand up straight, feet parallel, hip-width apart, shoulders down. Hold a weight in each hand in front of your thighs, palms facing back (see inset). Bend your knees as you hinge forwards from the hips, maintaining neutral spine alignment. The weights are now directly under your shoulders.

7b Inhale, then, as you exhale, raise your arms to the sides, in line with the shoulders, to shoulder height. Keep shoulder blades together as you lift your arms, elbows rounded, palms backwards. Inhale and lower your arms, then exhale as you straighten your hips and knees to return to start position (see inset, left). Repeat combination for 8 reps.

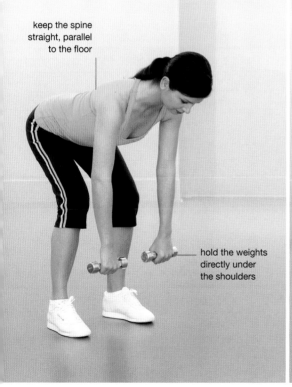

keep the spine straight, parallel to the floor

hold the weights directly under the shoulders

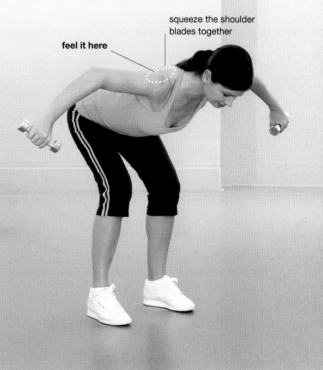

squeeze the shoulder blades together

feel it here

>> step-hop/jig

8 Put down the weights for the first cardio interval. Stand with your feet parallel, hip-width apart, arms by your sides. Step forwards with one leg and hop on it, as your raise the other knee to hip height. The arm opposite the raised leg swings forwards, elbow bent. Lower the leg and step back to the starting position. Alternate legs, swinging your arms in opposition, for a total of 6 reps (1 rep = both sides).

9 To begin, jump in place, feet hip width apart, hands on your hips. Hop on one leg, extending the other leg on a diagonal, digging your heel into the floor, toe pointing towards the ceiling. Bring the exended leg back and repeat on the other side. Keep your upper body vertical, chest lifted, eyes looking straight ahead. Alternate legs for a total of 8 reps (1 rep = both sides).

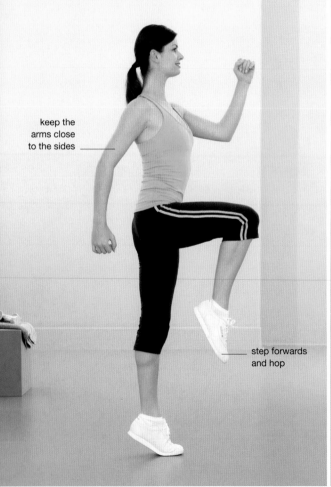

keep the arms close to the sides

step forwards and hop

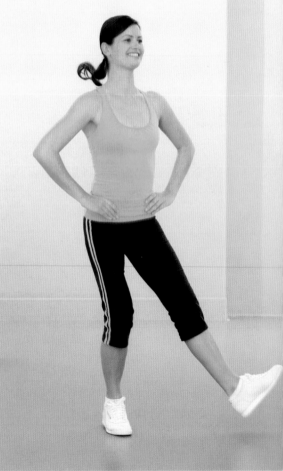

10 With your feet together, arms out to the sides, contract your abs and jump up, rotating your hips to one side. Turn your hips, knees, and feet as a unit. Land with your knees bent. Keep your torso upright, your shoulders facing forwards. Alternate sides for a total of 8 reps (1 rep = both sides). **Steps 8–10 complete your cardio interval, which you will repeat after each resistance exercise.**

11a Pick up one large free weight. Step forwards with one leg into a staggered lunge position. Hold the weight with both hands horizontally in front of your waist, elbows bent. Keep your weight centred between your legs, your back heel down and your feet parallel. Your shoulders should be square to the front, your eyes looking straight ahead.

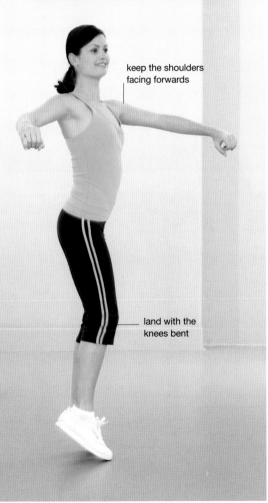

keep the shoulders facing forwards

land with the knees bent

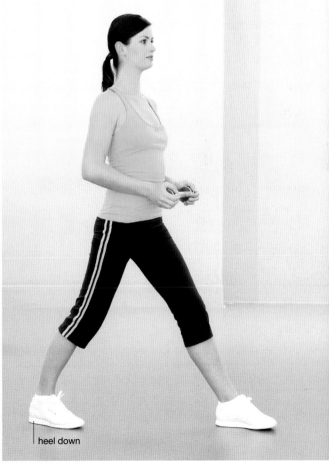

heel down

>> lunge and twist

11b Inhale as you bend both knees into a low lunge. Bend your front knee at a right angle directly over the ankle, the thigh parallel to the floor; bend your back knee close to the floor with the back heel lifted. As you come into the lunge, twist through your torso, reaching the weight towards your little toe. Keep your shoulder blades drawn together and your head and neck aligned with your spine, being careful not to round the upper back.

11c Exhale as you return to the starting position and then lift the weight high on a diagonal above your opposite shoulder, elbows bent. Keep looking forwards. Do 6 reps of the sequence, bending your knees into a lunge as you lower the weight before lifting it again. Switch sides for another 6 reps. **Then do your next cardio interval, steps 8–10 (pp192–193).**

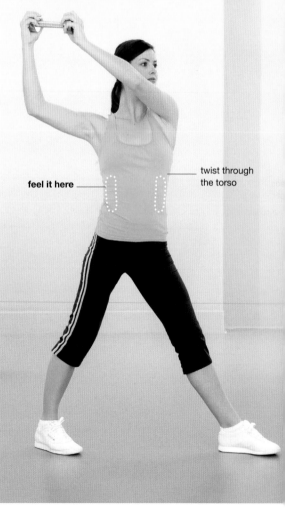

feel it here

twist through the torso

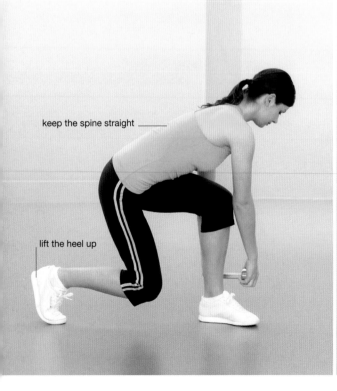

keep the spine straight

lift the heel up

>> side-squat/jump

12a Stand with your feet parallel, hip-width apart, knees soft, your hands on your hips. Step one leg to the side so that your feet are shoulder-width apart (see inset). Shift your weight back onto your heels as you bend your knees into a squat. Reach back with your hips, keeping your chest lifted.

12b Spring from both feet, jumping straight up. Land in a squat, knees bent, weight centred. Straighten your legs, step back to centre, and repeat, stepping to the other side. Do 4 reps (1 rep = both sides) for a total of 8 squats. **Do the next cardio interval, steps 8–10 (pp192–193).**

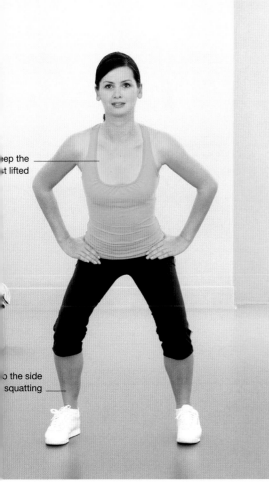

ep the
t lifted

o the side
squatting

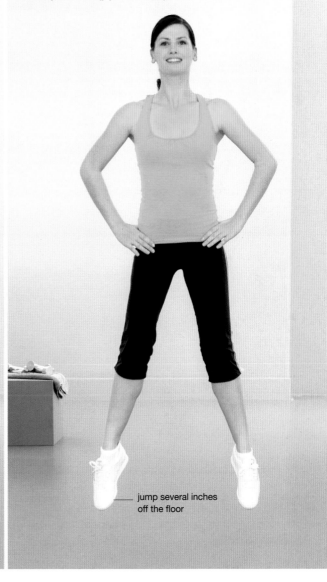

jump several inches
off the floor

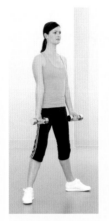

13 Stand with feet parallel, hip-width apart. Hold two small weights at shoulder height (see inset). Exhale, extending one arm, lifting opposite knee. Balance, inhale and step in place, alternating sides for 8 reps (1 rep = both sides). **Do your next cardio interval, steps 8–10 (pp192–193).**

14 Pick up two large weights, holding one in each hand. Stand in a wide stance, legs turned out to 45 degrees. Keep your arms by your sides (see inset). Inhale and bend your knees and elbows at the same time, lifting the weights towards your shoulders. Exhale as you straighten your arms and legs. **Do your next cardio interval, steps 8–10 (pp192–193).**

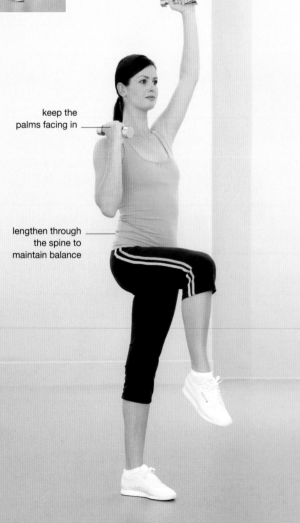

keep the palms facing in

lengthen through the spine to maintain balance

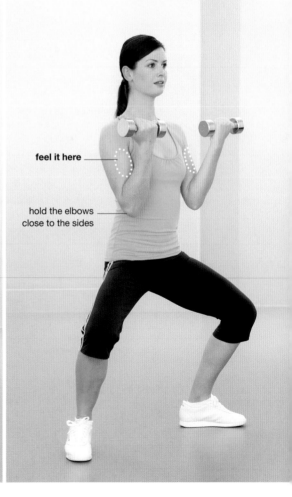

feel it here

hold the elbows close to the sides

15a Pick up two small weights. Stand with your feet parallel, hip-width apart, knees bent. Hold one weight in each hand, arms by your sides, palms facing inwards. Make sure your torso is aligned and ready for action: stack your ribs over your hips, engage the abs, draw your shoulder blades down, and lift your chest.

15b Inhale, then exhale as you straighten your legs, lifting one to the side, as you raise both arms to shoulder height, palms down. Your arms should be straight but not stiff. Inhale, then return to the starting position, bending the knees and squaring the hips. Alternate legs, lifting both arms every time for 12 reps (1 rep = both sides).

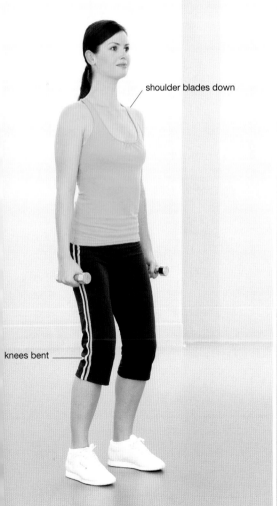

shoulder blades down

knees bent

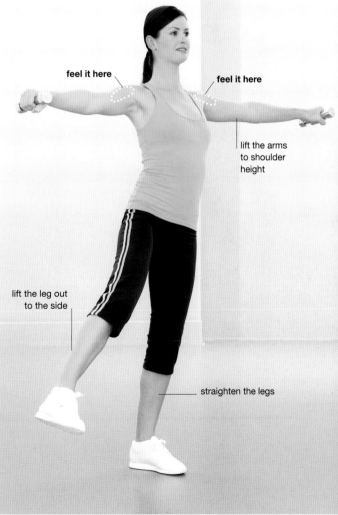

feel it here

feel it here

lift the arms to shoulder height

lift the leg out to the side

straighten the legs

>> flat back stretch/spinal twist

16 Get your mat for the cool down, and stand with your legs hip-width apart, hands on your hips. Lengthen through the spine, lifting the top of your head towards the ceiling. Draw your shoulder blades down and together. Bend forwards from your hips until your back is parallel to the floor, still elongating the spine by reaching your head forwards. Keep your knees straight, but not locked. Breathe deeply while you hold the stretch.

17 From the flat back position, reach one hand across your body to the opposite foot, and lift the other arm straight up to the ceiling, palm forwards. If you are able, press the heel of the supporting hand down on the mat. However, you may be more comfortable resting it on your ankle. Keep your knees straight and your hips level. Breathe naturally throughout, then swap sides and repeat.

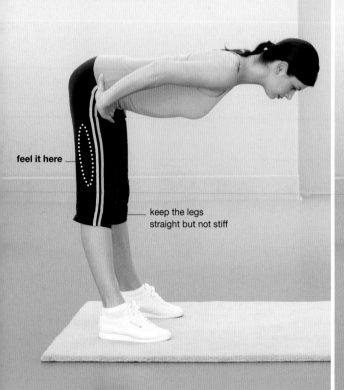

feel it here

keep the legs
straight but not stiff

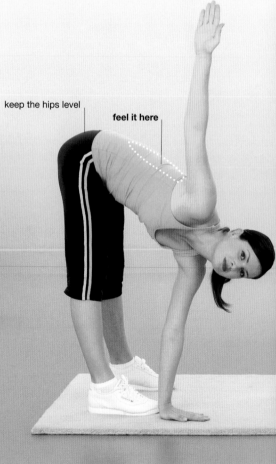

keep the hips level

feel it here

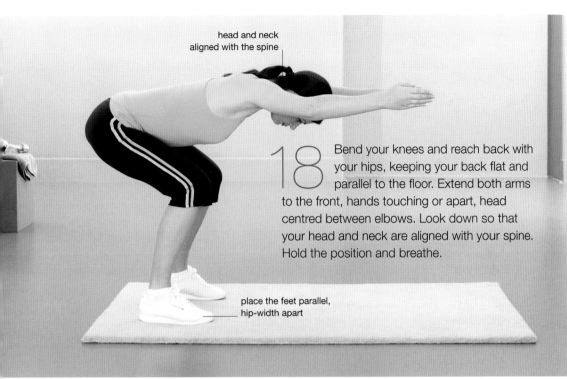

head and neck
aligned with the spine

18 Bend your knees and reach back with your hips, keeping your back flat and parallel to the floor. Extend both arms to the front, hands touching or apart, head centred between elbows. Look down so that your head and neck are aligned with your spine. Hold the position and breathe.

place the feet parallel,
hip-width apart

19 Kneel on all fours, wrists beneath shoulders, knees under hips. Lift one leg to the back, keeping the knee straight, then reach forwards with the opposite hand. Use deep breathing to increase the stretch, reaching further on every exhale.

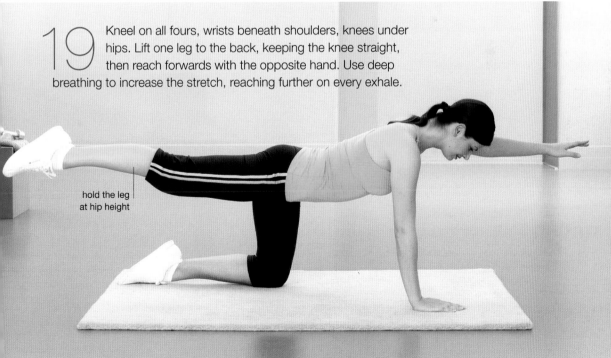

hold the leg
at hip height

>> calf stretch/spinal curve

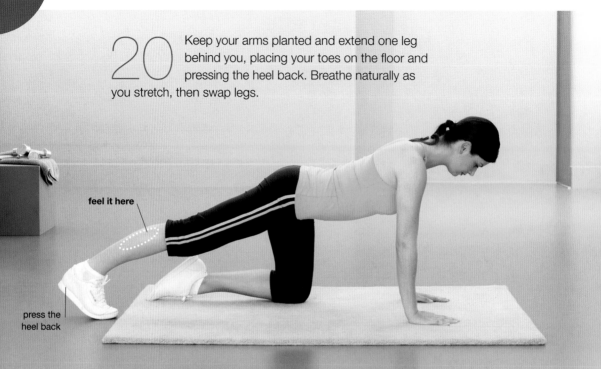

20 Keep your arms planted and extend one leg behind you, placing your toes on the floor and pressing the heel back. Breathe naturally as you stretch, then swap legs.

feel it here

press the
heel back

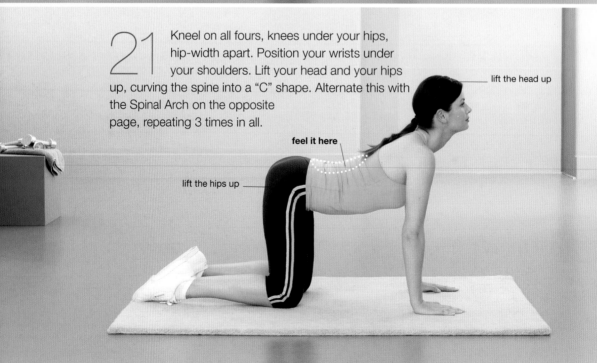

21 Kneel on all fours, knees under your hips, hip-width apart. Position your wrists under your shoulders. Lift your head and your hips up, curving the spine into a "C" shape. Alternate this with the Spinal Arch on the opposite page, repeating 3 times in all.

lift the head up

feel it here

lift the hips up

22 Start from a kneeling positon, knees under hips, wrists under shoulders, your back neutral. Then arch your spine, rounding it up to the ceiling by tucking your hips under and dropping your head between your arms. Alternate this with Spinal Curve (see 21, opposite), repeating 3 times in all.

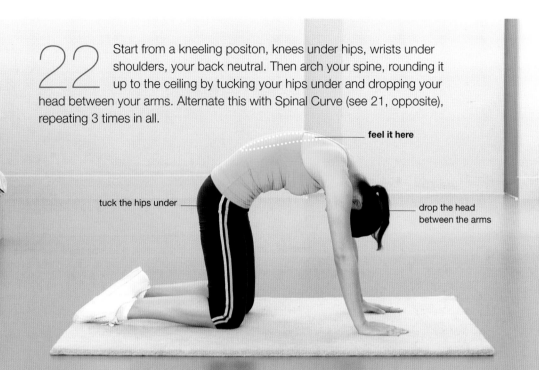

feel it here

tuck the hips under

drop the head between the arms

23 Sit back, reaching your hips towards your heels, at the same time rounding forward and extending your arms in front of you until your head rests on the mat. Keep your elbows off the mat to get the best stretch. Sink down into the position, holding for 3 deep breathing cycles, and sinking deeper into the position with each exhalation to complete your cool down.

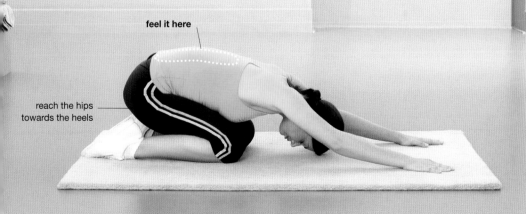

feel it here

reach the hips towards the heels

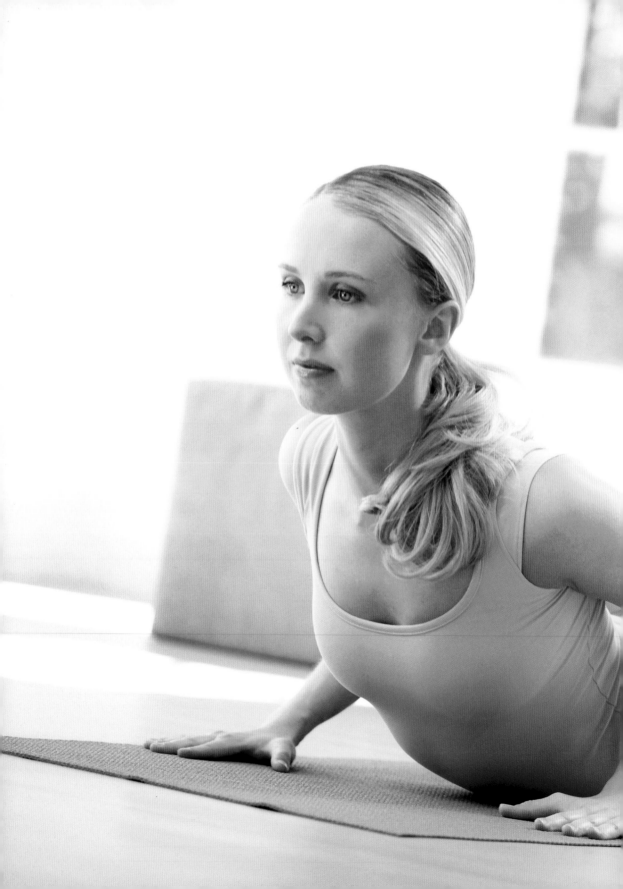

>> **15** minute

gentle
yoga

Louise Grime

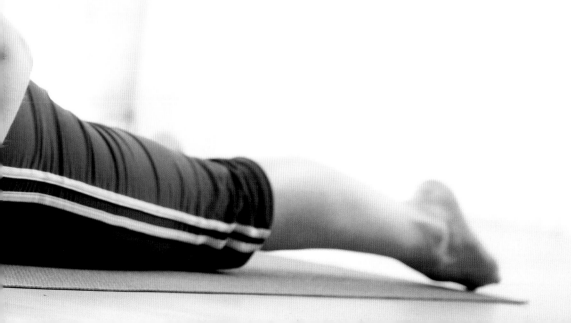

>> yoga for everyone

Welcome to yoga, whether you are trying it out to feel fitter and more flexible, or to destress and energize your mind and body. As you practise, you may find that yoga becomes a way of life and you start to approach every aspect of your day with an inquiring, balanced yoga mind-set.

When you embrace yoga, it becomes much more than what you do on the mat – it begins to filter into your way of thinking and interacting with others. As the postures and breathing practices make you feel bright and alive, so your self-confidence and energy levels soar. As you begin to notice where in the body you hold tension, and free it up by stretching and breathing more effectively, so you begin to become less stressed in your mind, too, and more able to appreciate life from different perspectives – just as yoga postures ask you to see the world upside down, backwards, or sideways on. As your physical balance improves, so does your ability to adopt a more measured approach to decision-making and problem-solving, enhancing every aspect of life, from your relationships at home and work to the way in which you do business. Above all, yoking together your body and mind with the single focus of a yoga posture makes every part of you feel more harmonious.

What is hatha yoga?

In the West, people tend to think of yoga as a system of physical exercises (known as *asanas*) and breathing techniques (known as *pranayama*). But this type of yoga – *hatha* yoga – is simply one route towards the ultimate aim of yoga, which is to feel so profoundly at peace within that we become aware of a connection with all the other elements in the universe. In India, where yoga originated many thousands of years ago, people follow other yoga paths to the same end-state of harmonious union:

>> weaving yoga into your life

- **Try to joyfully accept** your current physical limitations. Learn to work with stiff hamstrings or tight shoulders, rather than struggle against them, and you'll become more adept more quickly.

- **Don't be dispirited** when you first begin yoga. Keep a sense of humour, and be kind to your body, and the knots in your mind will also start to unwind.

- **Be patient and watch your breath** rather than pushing yourself to compete, and soon you will experience the bliss of yoga.

bhakti yoga, the path of religious worship; *karma* yoga, doing selfless service for others (Mother Teresa epitomizes this path of yoga); *jnana* yoga, studying yogic philosophy; and *raja* yoga, meditation. Each of these yoga paths suits a different personality type. You have probably turned to *hatha* yoga, the physical aspect of yoga, because, like many people in the West, you are interested in boosting your health and well-being, and would like to achieve a little more inner peace. As you clean and loosen out your body with its postures, you taste the lightness of being that is *hatha* yoga.

Finding a teacher

When you practise yoga with a teacher, you gain expert advice, as well as invaluable hands-on adjustments. Working with a teacher also helps you to gain the confidence to progress to more difficult poses and to work with breathing and meditation techniques. If you attend a regular yoga class, you will also build up a network of supportive fellow students to help you to maintain motivation.

But how do you find a teacher to suit you, and a style of yoga from the many confusing options on offer? The best way is to visit a yoga centre or gym close to your home or workplace. You can also look for local classes on notice boards in your doctors' surgery and library, for example. Ask for a list of classes and a description of the style of class if it is not a general "hatha yoga" class (which may draw on a mix of styles – *hatha* yoga can be taught in myriad ways). Iyengar yoga, the most practised form of yoga across the globe, focuses on alignment and precision in the physical postures using props such as blocks and belts, and offers a sound foundation for beginners. If you enjoy fast-moving exercise, you might try *Ashtanga vinyasa* classes, which teach a seamless flow of postures (classes might be called *vinyasa* flow, dynamic or power yoga). If you prefer a more esoteric approach that includes chanting and a focus on breathing, meditation and energy-raising techniques, look out for Sivananda or Kundalini yoga. If you have an on-going health problem, try therapeutic Iyengar yoga or Viniyoga, which tailors sequences of poses to suit your particular healing needs. If you are pregnant or post-natal, find a class especially geared for you. What's important is that you find the teacher inspiring and approachable. In the end this matters more than the type of yoga you follow.

A teacher offers hands-on adjustments while you hold a pose, which help you to relax effortlessly into the posture and to let go of held-in tension.

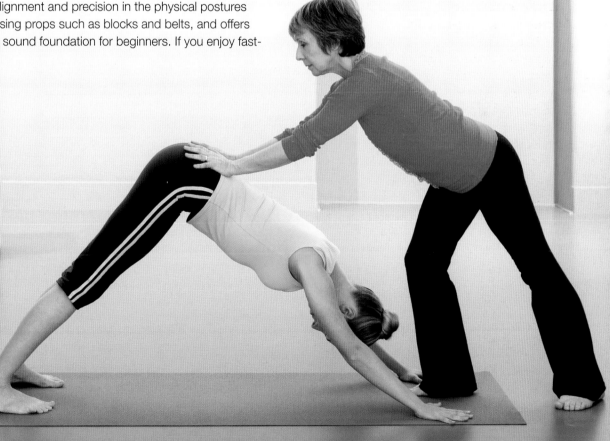

>> **advice** for beginners

Once you are on your mat, following the sequences set out in this book, you'll find the 15 minutes fly by as you focus on getting to know your body and mind better. What is more tricky is maintaining the enthusiasm and motivation to roll out the mat in the first place. These tips may help.

The most important advice a teacher can offer beginners to yoga is to make the time to roll out their mats. Practising in the same place and at the same time can help maintain motivation. Decide on a time and write it into your diary, thinking of it as an appointment you cannot miss. Indeed, this may be one of the most important appointments you make during a day since it allows you to devote time to looking after yourself. This not only makes you feel great, it sets you up for success in every other part of your day, whether that includes achieving work tasks or mixing with other people.

Setting practice times

Early morning is traditionally considered the best time of day to practise yoga. Try setting your alarm 30 minutes earlier than usual. Take a shower and then practise in the quiet period before the rest of your household awakes. It is interesting to note how this period of reflection first thing can make your home life feel less stressed.

Late afternoon or early evening make good alternative practice times, especially if you need an energy boost or would like to wind down after a hectic day. Wash before you begin and make sure your stomach is empty: let two hours pass after a meal before you practise.

Planning the session

At the start of any yoga session, spend a few minutes sitting, or lying on your back with your knees bent and feet flat on the floor. Close your

>> **before** you begin

- **Remove your watch**, glasses and any jewellery that might get in the way of your practice. If you have long hair, tie it back.

- **Gather together your props**, which may include a belt and yoga blocks, a chair or bolsters, plus a blanket to keep you warm in the final relaxation pose.

- **Turn off your phone**, and any other sensory distractions, such as the radio or music.

- **Close the door** and make sure those who share your home know not to disturb you.

eyes and look inside yourself, watching your breath flow in and out completely naturally. Then carefully follow the warm-up exercises before beginning the postures. Allow at least five minutes after finishing the routine to lie in the final relaxation pose that ends all yoga sessions.

Take it slowly

Yoga is all about getting to know your capabilities and limitations – but you have the rest of your life to complete this study. Do not feel pressured to push it too far or too fast in the early weeks and months, and do let go of any thoughts of perfection. Yoga is not competitive.

Follow your breath

Tune into your breath not only at the beginning of each session, but in every posture to see what it tells you about your practice. If your breathing becomes ragged or uneven at any time take it as a sign to ease off a little. When you arrive in a pose, explore whether breathing out any tension makes you feel more comfortable, and whether the in-breath allows you to expand and reach a little further. With time, breath-awareness will become second-nature.

Listen to your body

Honour the messages your body sends. If your knees or lower back hurt, for example, take it as an instruction to refer to the easier version of the posture. Acknowledge your limitations, taking things slowly and not progressing to the stronger stretches in the sequences until fully ready – but do not accept your current limitations as your fate. Yoga encourages us to explore the boundaries of what we can do, and to challenge ourselves, but without pursuing perfection, which may lead to physical injury and to unhelpful emotions such as anger or pride. The key to a fulfilling yoga practice is to let expectations go, but to keep pushing into your "edges". Try to incorporate some yoga poses into your everyday life, for example, practise leg raises while you are on the phone or sit on the floor with your back straight while you are reading or watching television, instead of slouching on the sofa, and you will soon notice a real difference.

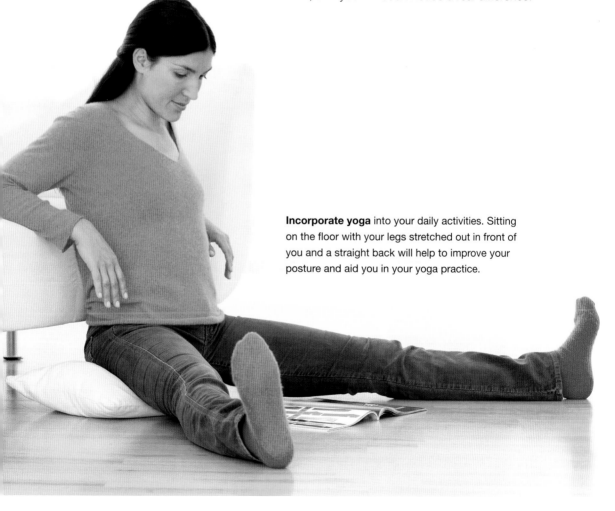

Incorporate yoga into your daily activities. Sitting on the floor with your legs stretched out in front of you and a straight back will help to improve your posture and aid you in your yoga practice.

>> **practising** safely

Yoga is about knowing yourself. It is important not to push your body beyond its limits. If some of the postures are difficult to start with, feel pleased that you have a challenge ahead of you. For more difficult poses, there are easier options throughout the book for you to refer to.

If you are not used to doing exercise, it is important that you learn the difference between sweet pain – a good, stretchy feeling in the muscles – and sour, or negative, pain – a sharp or nagging pain. This can take time to understand; go slowly.

To begin with, you may feel some stiffness for a day or two afterwards, but this will soon pass. Do not force your body into positions that it cannot perform. If you find that a pose creates negative pain or tension in a part of your body, ease off. Always veer on the safe side and modify the pose, referring to the easier option for positions that cause you difficulty.

Always practise yoga on an empty stomach. Allow two to three hours to elapse after a meal before starting yoga.

If you have a specific injury, are pregnant or have any other health concerns, consult a doctor before using this book. If you feel dizzy, experience chest pain or heart irregularity, or become short of breath while practising yoga, stop immediately.

Use your environment to help you. Use a shelf for support for a modified standing bend instead of Downward Dog (p215) and a wall or door to lean your legs up against at the end of a tiring day.

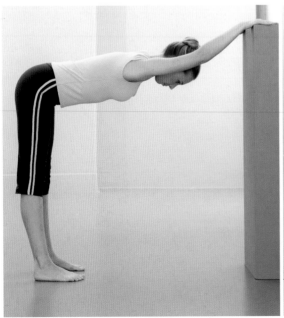
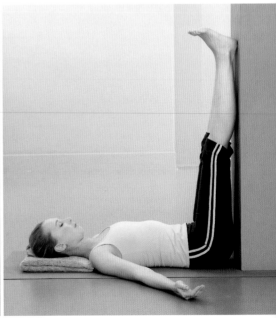

>> **before** you begin

- **Consult** a doctor before practising yoga if you have an injury, any health concerns, or you are pregnant.

- **Practise** on an empty stomach. Allow three hours to pass after a large meal, two hours after a light meal, and one hour after a snack.

- **Do not over-reach** yourself. Take it slowly at first and stop if you are experiencing any negative pain or tension.

- **Refer to the easier options** where relevant and use props to help you in difficult poses.

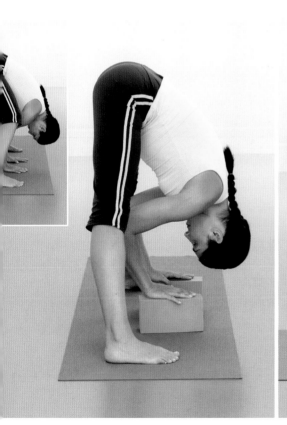

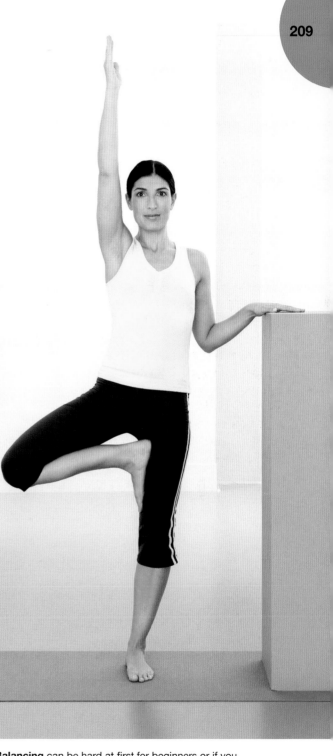

you find it difficult to reach the floor in a standing forward bend, bend your knees (see inset) or place a block under your hands.

Balancing can be hard at first for beginners or if you are feeling particularly tired. Use a wall to lean against or a surface to hold on to.

15 minute

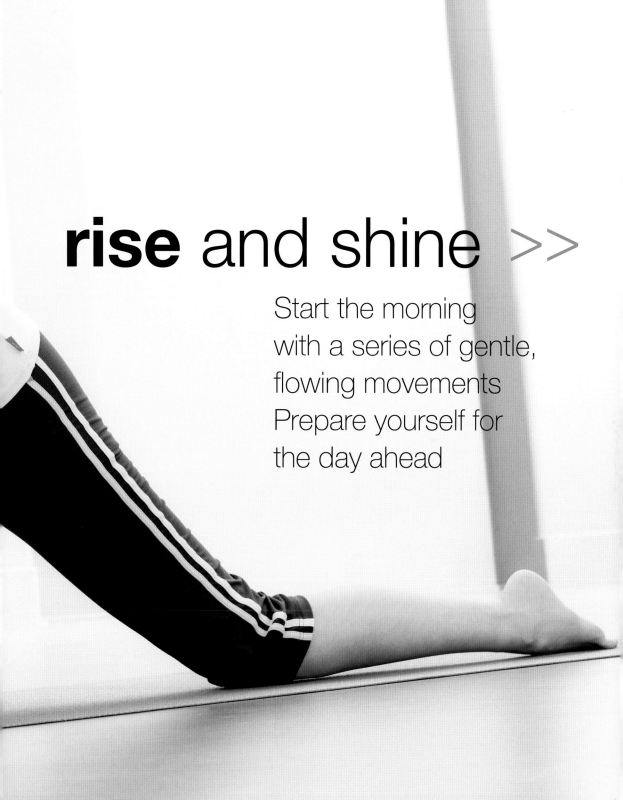

rise and shine >>

Start the morning
with a series of gentle,
flowing movements
Prepare yourself for
the day ahead

>> **listening to your breath**

1 Lie flat on your back with your knees bent and your arms out at 45 degrees to your body. Keep the back of your neck long. Close your eyes and listen to your natural breath coming and going. To bring more awareness into your lungs, breathe in steadily for 3 counts and out for 4, repeating several times.

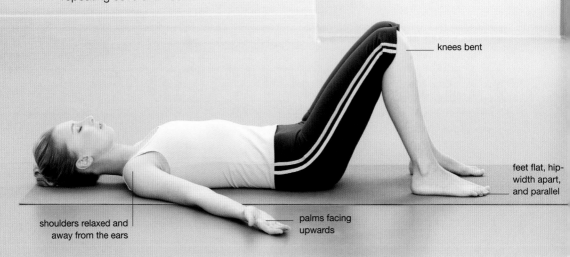

knees bent

feet flat, hip-width apart, and parallel

shoulders relaxed and away from the ears

palms facing upwards

2 Inhale and bend your knees towards your chest, with your hands resting on your knees. Keep the back of your neck long.

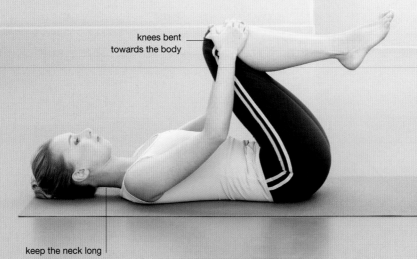

knees bent towards the body

keep the neck long

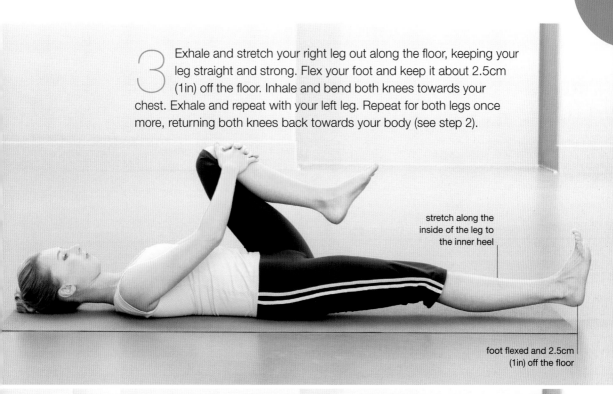

3 Exhale and stretch your right leg out along the floor, keeping your leg straight and strong. Flex your foot and keep it about 2.5cm (1in) off the floor. Inhale and bend both knees towards your chest. Exhale and repeat with your left leg. Repeat for both legs once more, returning both knees back towards your body (see step 2).

stretch along the inside of the leg to the inner heel

foot flexed and 2.5cm (1in) off the floor

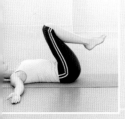

4 Keep your knees bent towards your chest and stretch your arms out to your sides. Exhale and take both knees down towards your right elbow. At the same time, turn your head and abdomen towards the left. Inhale and come back to the centre (see inset). Exhale and repeat on your left side, as you turn your head and navel towards the right. Repeat on both sides, returning to the centre each time.

head and abdomen turned away from your knees

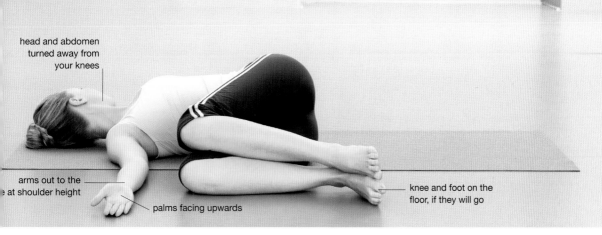

arms out to the side at shoulder height

palms facing upwards

knee and foot on the floor, if they will go

>> rock and roll/circling

5 Start to awaken the spine. With your knees still hugged towards your body, but holding the back of your knees, gently rock backwards and forwards on your spine. Inhale as you roll back. Exhale as you roll forward. Repeat several times. If your back feels too stiff, just roll gently from side-to-side instead.

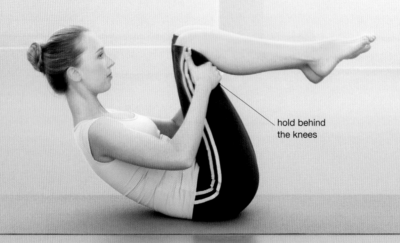

hold behind
the knees

6 Turn to the side to come onto all-fours, facing the front of the mat. Your hands shoulder-width apart, facing forward, and your knees are hip-width apart with the tops of your feet flat on the floor. Circle your hips 3 times to the left, taking one full breath for each circle. Feel like you are drawing a circle with your navel out to your hips. Repeat to the right. Feel your lower back relaxing.

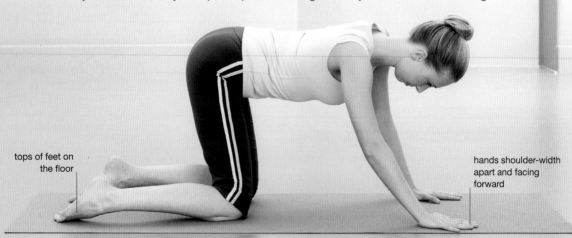

tops of feet on
the floor

hands shoulder-width
apart and facing
forward

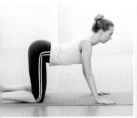

7 Inhale and look ahead. Keep your shoulders away from your ears and your tailbone back (see inset). Exhale, rounding your back down and looking to your navel, as you stretch your buttocks and down towards your heels, with your head resting on the floor for Child's Pose. Your hands are on the floor in front of you. At first, your head may not touch the floor and your buttocks may not reach your heels. If your knees feel very stiff, place a blanket behind the knees. If your ankles hurt, place a rolled towel under them.

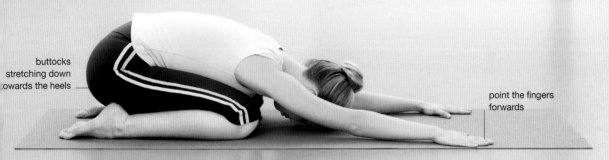

buttocks stretching down towards the heels

point the fingers forwards

easier option

push the sitting bones up

8 Inhale and come up onto all-fours again, placing your feet flat on the floor. Look ahead. Keep your shoulders away from your ears and draw your navel back to the spine. Exhale and tuck your toes under, as you come up into Downward Dog. Push away and down with your heels and up with your buttocks, lengthening your spine. Bend your knees if your hamstrings feel too tight (see inset). Repeat steps 7–8 once more.

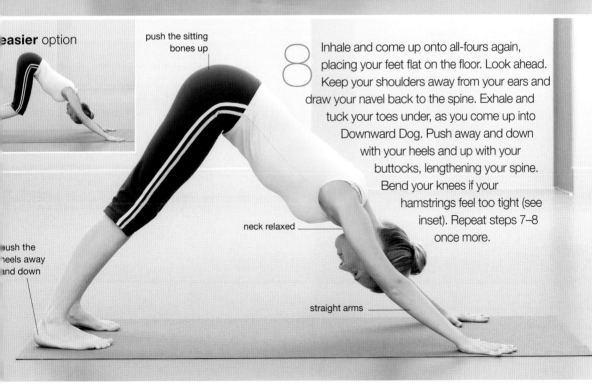

push the heels away and down

neck relaxed

straight arms

9 Gently walk your feet and hands towards each other until you are in a Standing Forward Bend. Your feet are parallel and hip-width apart. If your back feels stiff, keep your legs bent (see inset). Inhale, bending your knees more. Exhale, lifting your kneecaps and sucking the front of your thighs up and back. Feel your feet growing roots down into the floor, relaxed, but grounding down. Breathe freely.

easier option

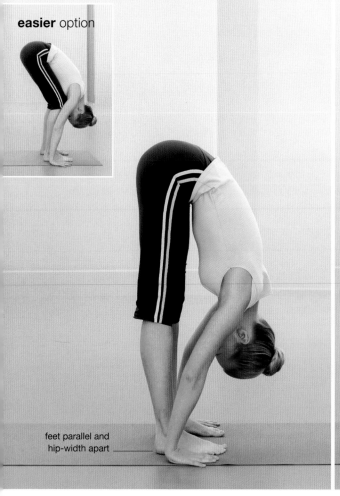

feet parallel and hip-width apart

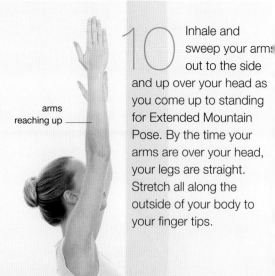

arms reaching up

10 Inhale and sweep your arms out to the side and up over your head as you come up to standing for Extended Mountain Pose. By the time your arms are over your head, your legs are straight. Stretch all along the outside of your body to your finger tips.

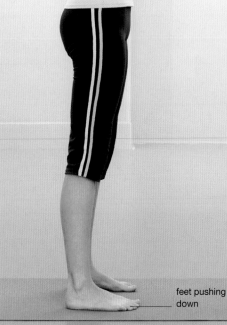

feet pushing down

11 Exhale, bringing your arms out and down by your side. Step your feet together at the front of the mat and stand in Mountain Pose. Feel a plumb line through the centre of your body. Get ready for 2 rounds of Sun Salutation.

12 Exhale and bring your hands into Prayer Position in front of your chest. Inhale and sweep your arms out and up over your head (see inset). Look up.

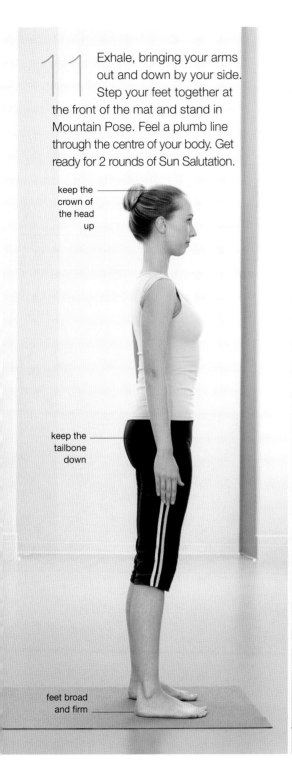

keep the crown of the head up

keep the tailbone down

feet broad and firm

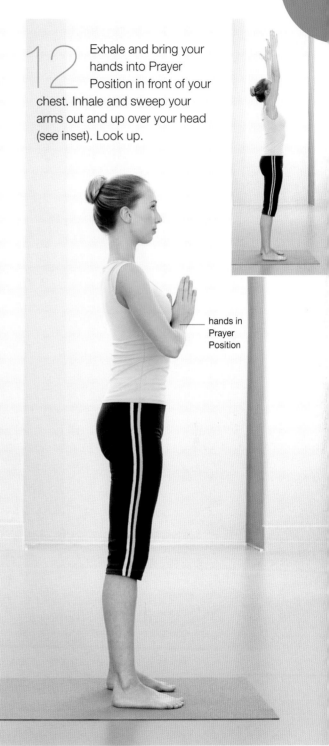

hands in Prayer Position

>> forward bend/lunge

13 Exhale and swing your arms out and down as you bend forward into Standing Forward Bend. Place your hands on the floor by the side of your feet, but allow your knees to bend if necessary. Keep your head relaxed.

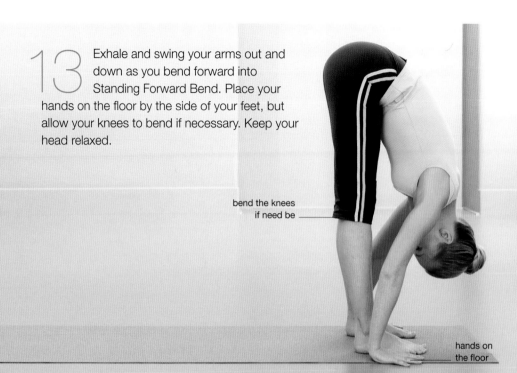

bend the knees if need be

hands on the floor

14 Inhale and bring your right leg back and your knee to the floor. Place your hands on the floor on either side of your front foot for a Lunge.

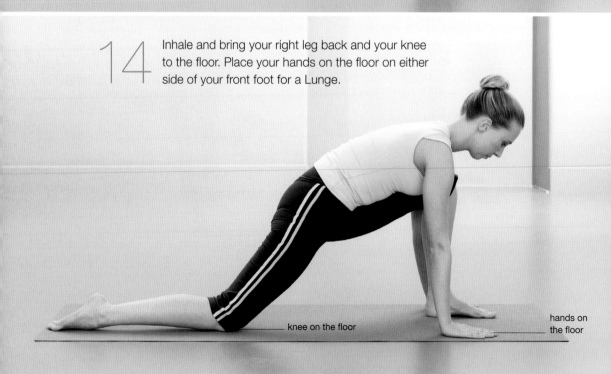

knee on the floor

hands on the floor

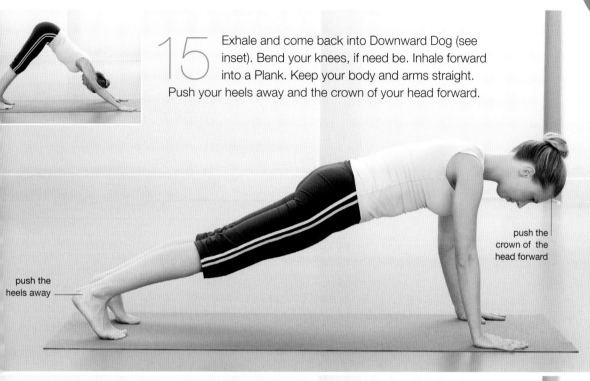

15 Exhale and come back into Downward Dog (see inset). Bend your knees, if need be. Inhale forward into a Plank. Keep your body and arms straight. Push your heels away and the crown of your head forward.

push the crown of the head forward

push the heels away

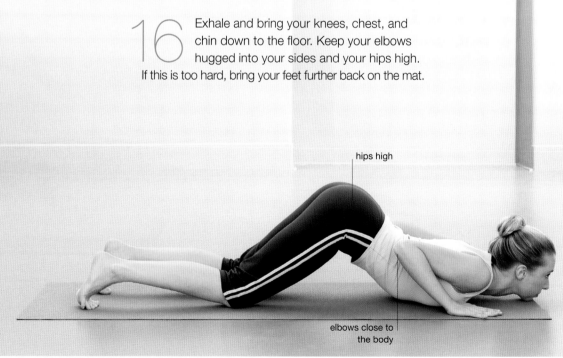

16 Exhale and bring your knees, chest, and chin down to the floor. Keep your elbows hugged into your sides and your hips high. If this is too hard, bring your feet further back on the mat.

hips high

elbows close to the body

>> cobra/downward dog

17 Inhale into the Cobra. Keep your elbows hugged into your sides and bring the tops of your feet and legs down onto the floor. Lengthen all along your legs to the inner heel. Push down with your pubic bone and lift your navel to your chest. Keep your shoulders down, away from your ears. Lift upwards with the top of your chest. Look ahead. If this is difficult, place your elbows and forearms on the floor in front of you for the Sphinx (see inset).

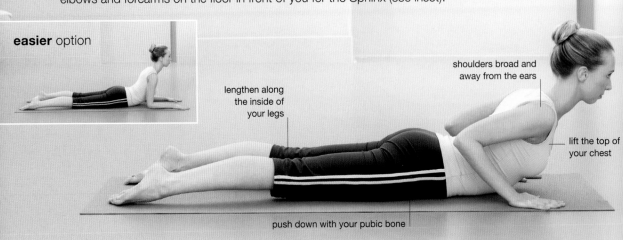

easier option

lengthen along the inside of your legs

shoulders broad and away from the ears

lift the top of your chest

push down with your pubic bone

18 Exhale and tuck your toes under and push up into the Downward Dog. Take a couple of breaths here. Inhale and bring your right foot forward, in between your hands, as you bring your left knee to the floor (see inset). Look ahead. If this is difficult, use your hand to bring the foot forward (see easier option).

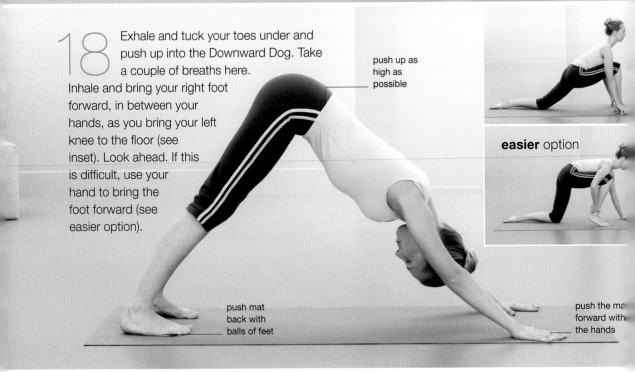

push up as high as possible

easier option

push mat back with balls of feet

push the ma[t] forward with the hands

19 Exhale and bring your back foot forward to join your front foot. Place your hands on the floor on either side of your feet for a Standing Forward Bend, keeping your knees bent if necessary. Keep your heels firm on the floor, but bring your weight further forward, so that you can feel your front thigh muscles lifting, the backs of your knees opening, and your calves stretching down to your heels.

20 Sweep your arms out to the side and up over your head as you come back up to standing. Look up. Exhale and bring your hands down the centre line to the chest into Prayer Position (see inset). Look ahead. Repeat steps 12–20 on your left side to complete one full round of the Sun Salutation, and then repeat another full round. Bring your hands down by the side of your body for Mountain Pose. Listen to your breath coming and going. Step back to the middle of the mat.

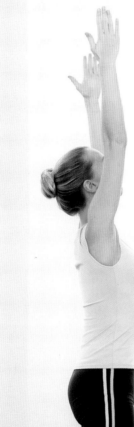

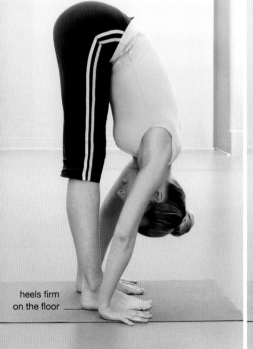

heels firm on the floor

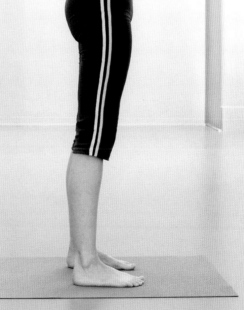

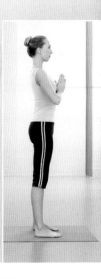

>> child's pose/lion

21 Kneel down to Child's Pose. Allow your big toes to touch, but keep your heels apart. Rest your forehead on the floor and let your sitting bones sink down to your heels. Bring your arms by your feet, palms facing upwards. Breathe naturally. As you inhale, you may feel your breath moving in your lower back. Exhale and relax.

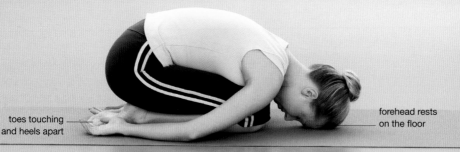

toes touching
and heels apart

forehead rests
on the floor

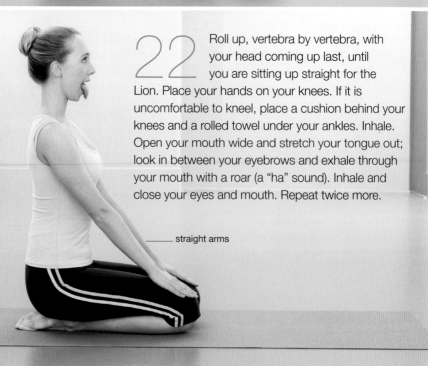

22 Roll up, vertebra by vertebra, with your head coming up last, until you are sitting up straight for the Lion. Place your hands on your knees. If it is uncomfortable to kneel, place a cushion behind your knees and a rolled towel under your ankles. Inhale. Open your mouth wide and stretch your tongue out; look in between your eyebrows and exhale through your mouth with a roar (a "ha" sound). Inhale and close your eyes and mouth. Repeat twice more.

straight arms

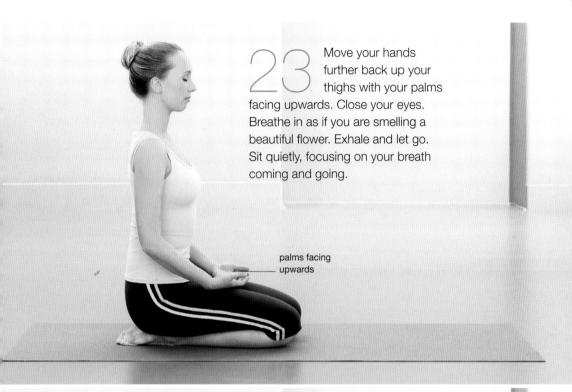

23 Move your hands further back up your thighs with your palms facing upwards. Close your eyes. Breathe in as if you are smelling a beautiful flower. Exhale and let go. Sit quietly, focusing on your breath coming and going.

palms facing upwards

24 Lie on your back with your knees bent and your feet flat on the floor (hip-width apart and parallel). Lift your head and look down your centre line to see that you are straight. Place your head on the floor and your arms away from your body. Lengthen one leg out along the floor and then the other, ready for the final relaxation. Stay here for 2–5 minutes. Place a folded blanket under your head, a cushion under your knees and an eye pad on your eyes, if you wish, to make you more comfortable.

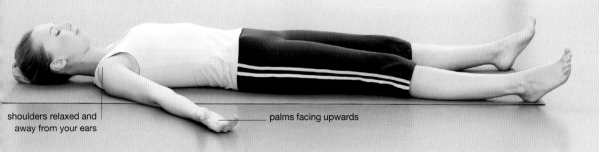

shoulders relaxed and away from your ears

palms facing upwards

15 minute

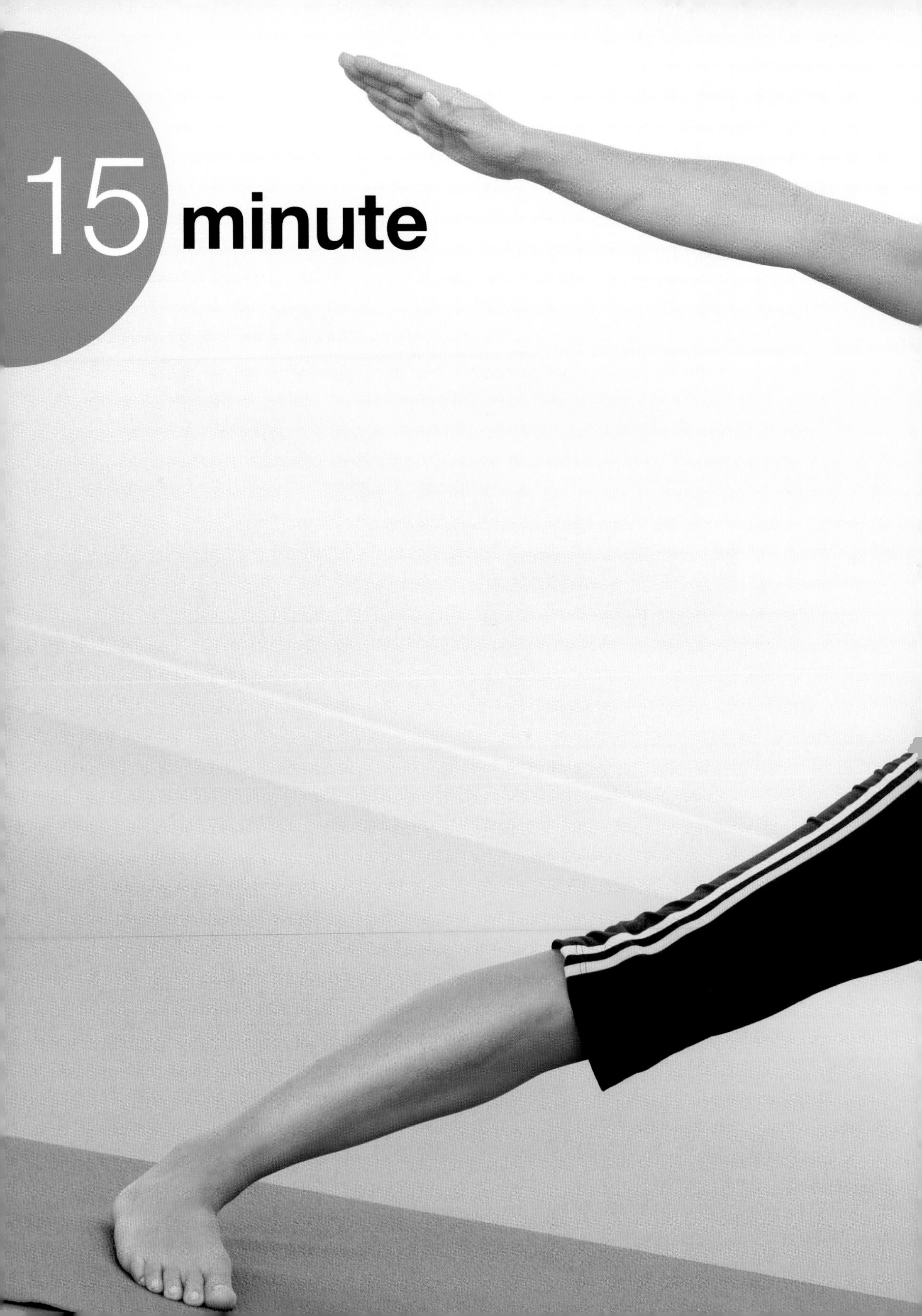

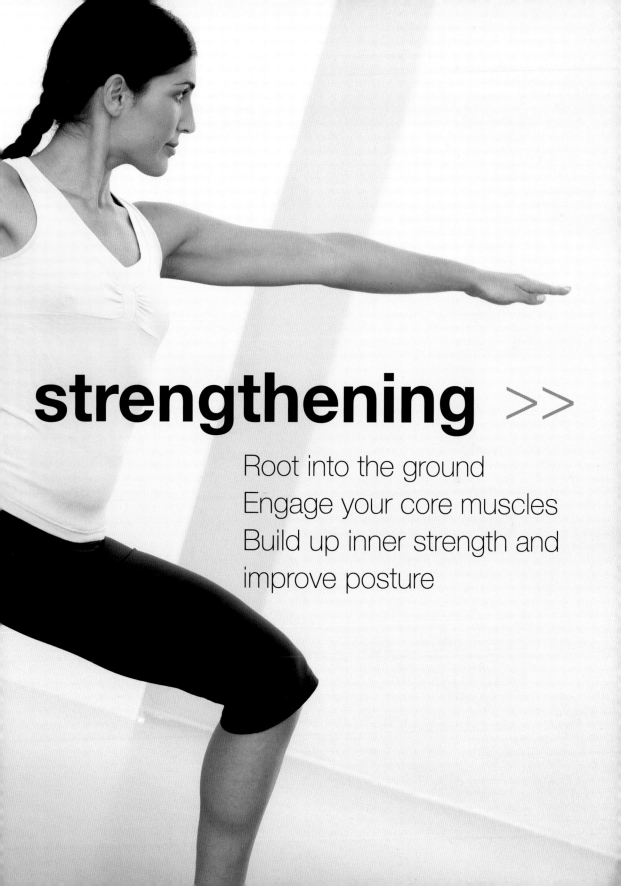

strengthening >>

Root into the ground
Engage your core muscles
Build up inner strength and
improve posture

>> **quieting the mind/shining skull**

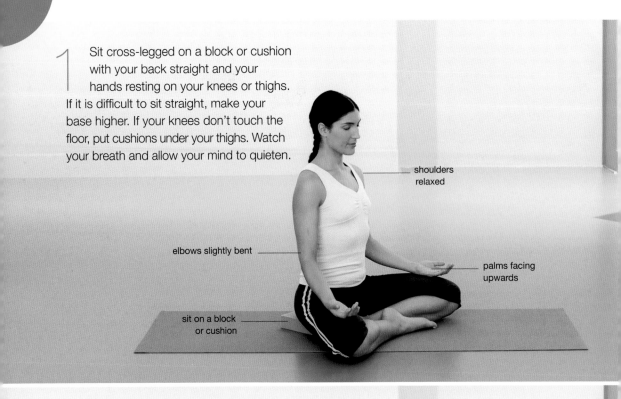

1 Sit cross-legged on a block or cushion with your back straight and your hands resting on your knees or thighs. If it is difficult to sit straight, make your base higher. If your knees don't touch the floor, put cushions under your thighs. Watch your breath and allow your mind to quieten.

shoulders relaxed

elbows slightly bent

palms facing upwards

sit on a block or cushion

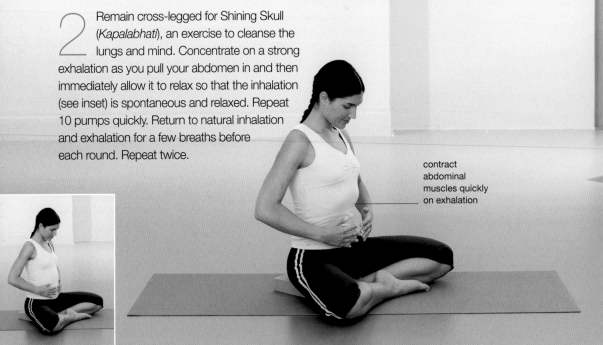

2 Remain cross-legged for Shining Skull (*Kapalabhati*), an exercise to cleanse the lungs and mind. Concentrate on a strong exhalation as you pull your abdomen in and then immediately allow it to relax so that the inhalation (see inset) is spontaneous and relaxed. Repeat 10 pumps quickly. Return to natural inhalation and exhalation for a few breaths before each round. Repeat twice.

contract abdominal muscles quickly on exhalation

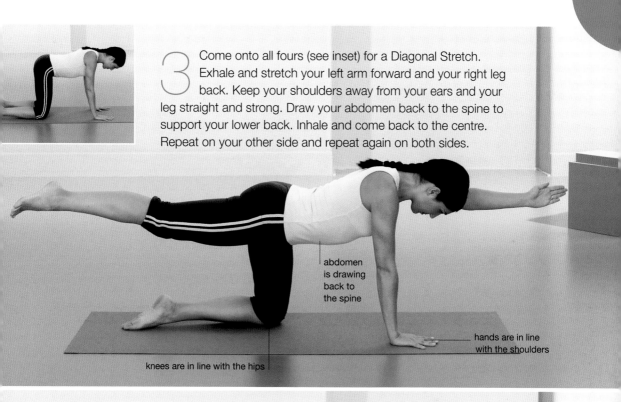

3 Come onto all fours (see inset) for a Diagonal Stretch. Exhale and stretch your left arm forward and your right leg back. Keep your shoulders away from your ears and your leg straight and strong. Draw your abdomen back to the spine to support your lower back. Inhale and come back to the centre. Repeat on your other side and repeat again on both sides.

abdomen is drawing back to the spine

hands are in line with the shoulders

knees are in line with the hips

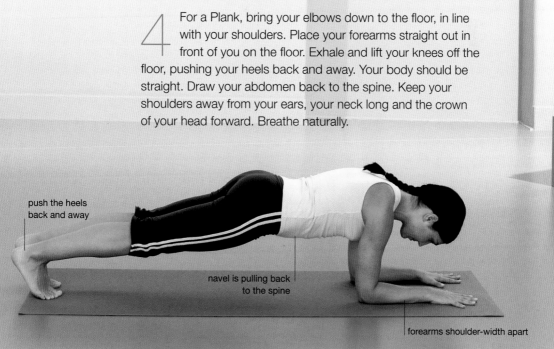

4 For a Plank, bring your elbows down to the floor, in line with your shoulders. Place your forearms straight out in front of you on the floor. Exhale and lift your knees off the floor, pushing your heels back and away. Your body should be straight. Draw your abdomen back to the spine. Keep your shoulders away from your ears, your neck long and the crown of your head forward. Breathe naturally.

push the heels back and away

navel is pulling back to the spine

forearms shoulder-width apart

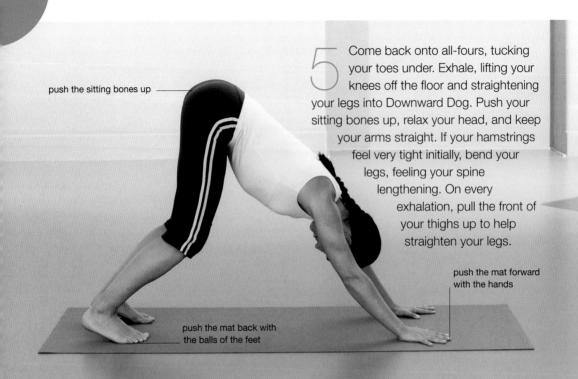

push the sitting bones up

5 Come back onto all-fours, tucking your toes under. Exhale, lifting your knees off the floor and straightening your legs into Downward Dog. Push your sitting bones up, relax your head, and keep your arms straight. If your hamstrings feel very tight initially, bend your legs, feeling your spine lengthening. On every exhalation, pull the front of your thighs up to help straighten your legs.

push the mat forward with the hands

push the mat back with the balls of the feet

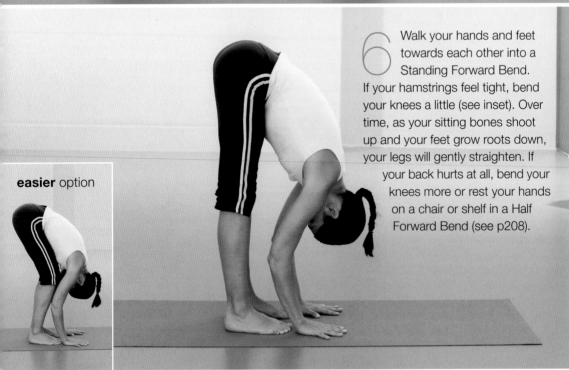

6 Walk your hands and feet towards each other into a Standing Forward Bend. If your hamstrings feel tight, bend your knees a little (see inset). Over time, as your sitting bones shoot up and your feet grow roots down, your legs will gently straighten. If your back hurts at all, bend your knees more or rest your hands on a chair or shelf in a Half Forward Bend (see p208).

easier option

7 Roll up, vertebra by vertebra, until you are in Mountain Pose. Stand with your feet hip-width apart, growing roots down. Draw your abdomen back to the spine. Breathe through your nose, feeling your breath softly caressing the back of your throat.

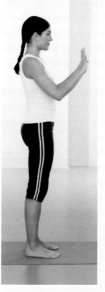

8 For the Tiptoes exercise, bring your hands in front of you at shoulder height with your palms facing forward and your elbows by your side. Inhale and come up onto the balls of your feet. Exhale and come down. Repeat 4 times.

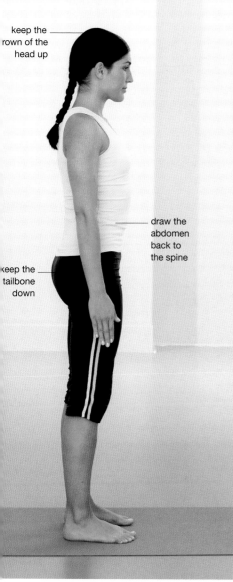

keep the crown of the head up

draw the abdomen back to the spine

keep the tailbone down

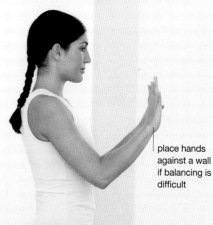

place hands against a wall if balancing is difficult

bring the heels up high as you come up onto tiptoes

>> chair pose/lateral stretch

9 Inhale and move your arms forward and up over your head as you come onto your tiptoes (see inset). Stretch up to your fingertips. Exhale, bringing your heels down, and bend your knees into the Chair Pose. Inhale, straightening your legs. Exhale, and bring your arms out and down by your side.

arms stay above the head for Chair Pose

10 Interlace your fingers for a Standing Lateral Stretch. Turn your hands out and push your palms away from you. Inhale, lifting your arms up over your head. Exhale, stretching to the right, with a firm weight on your left foot. Inhale back to the centre. Repeat to the left. Change the interlace of your fingers. Repeat once more on both sides.

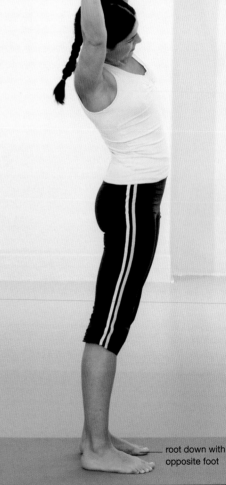

root down with opposite foot

11 Bring your arms out and down, ready for Standing Rhythmic Twist. With your knees slightly bent and your arms hanging loosely by your side, swing your upper body from left to right. Your arms are relaxed and gently swinging from side to side with your hands tapping your body. Breathe naturally as you rhythmically swing.

12 For Eagle Arms, lift your arms out to the side and wrap your right arm over your left. Place the fingers of your left hand into your right palm, and bring your thumbs in front of your nose. Push forward with your left hand and pull back with your right.

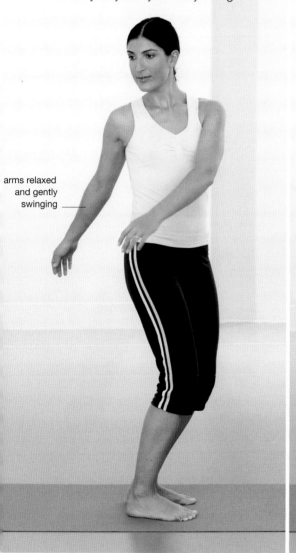

arms relaxed and gently swinging

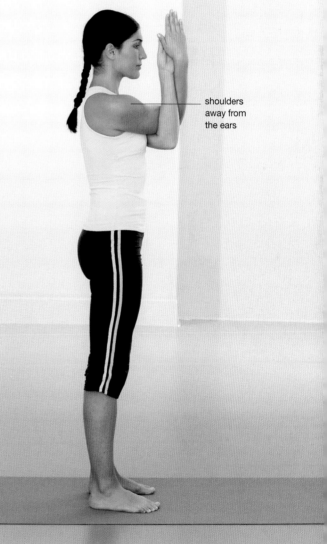

shoulders away from the ears

>> **squat/preparation for horse**

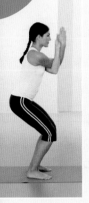

13 Exhale down into a Squat. Feel the weight on the outside of your feet. If it is difficult to squat, just come down as far as you are able, without lifting your heels (see inset). Inhale and come back up. Exhale and release your arms out to the side. Switch hands and repeat. Inhale and come up, releasing your arms out and down by your side.

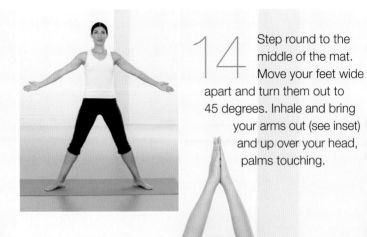

14 Step round to the middle of the mat. Move your feet wide apart and turn them out to 45 degrees. Inhale and bring your arms out (see inset) and up over your head, palms touching.

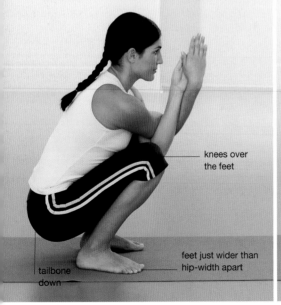

knees over the feet

feet just wider than hip-width apart

tailbone down

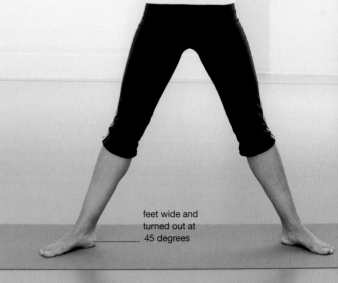

feet wide and turned out at 45 degrees

15 Exhale into the Horse, bending your knees so that they are in line with your feet and bringing your hands down through your centre line into Prayer Position. Inhale and push your feet into the floor to straighten your legs. Bring your arms over your head as you come up. Touch your palms together above your head. Repeat once more.

16 Inhale and straighten your legs. Stretch your arms out straight at shoulder height. Turn your right foot out and your left foot in for Triangle pose. Exhale out to the right, bringing your right hand to rest on your right shin, and your left arm up, straight. Inhale and look down at your front big toe. Exhale and look ahead. Take a couple of breaths here, come up, and repeat on the left side.

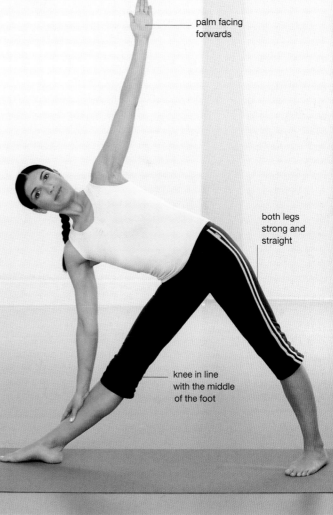

palm facing forwards

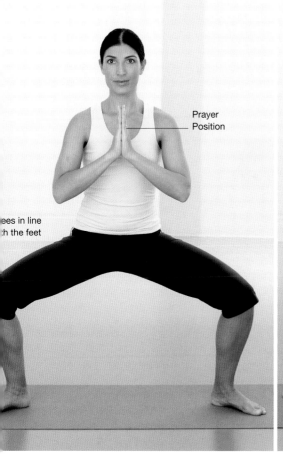

Prayer Position

both legs strong and straight

ees in line th the feet

knee in line with the middle of the foot

>> forward bend/warrior 2

17 Inhale and come back up to centre. For a Wide Leg Forward Bend, rest your hands on your hips. Inhale and look up. Exhale and hinge at your hips, bringing your hands down to the floor. Bend your knees a little, if need be, or use blocks to rest your hands on (see p209, bottom left picture). Walk your feet a little wider apart. Inhale and look ahead. Exhale, let your head go, and bring your hands further back, in line with your toes (see inset). Inhale and look ahead. Exhale and bring your hands to your hips. Inhale and come up.

feet parallel

hands in line with the shoulders

18 Turn your right foot out and keep your left foot in, ready for Warrior 2. Exhale and bend your right knee directly over your ankle. Rotate both your knees away from each other. Keep strong and straight on your left leg all the way to the outside of your foot. Inhale and stretch your arms out, looking out towards your right index finger. Have a couple of breaths here.

arms out at shoulder height

the calf forms a right angle with the thigh

rotate the knee out

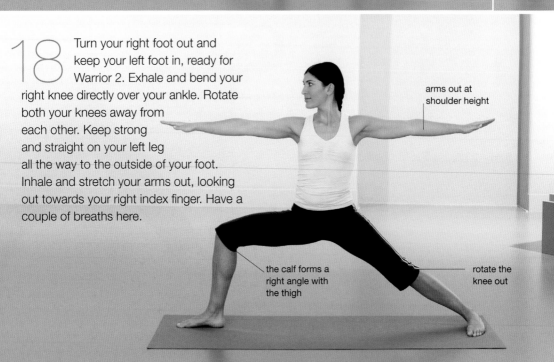

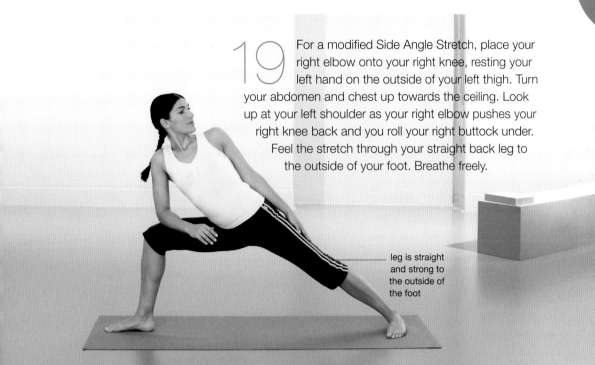

19 For a modified Side Angle Stretch, place your right elbow onto your right knee, resting your left hand on the outside of your left thigh. Turn your abdomen and chest up towards the ceiling. Look up at your left shoulder as your right elbow pushes your right knee back and you roll your right buttock under. Feel the stretch through your straight back leg to the outside of your foot. Breathe freely.

leg is straight and strong to the outside of the foot

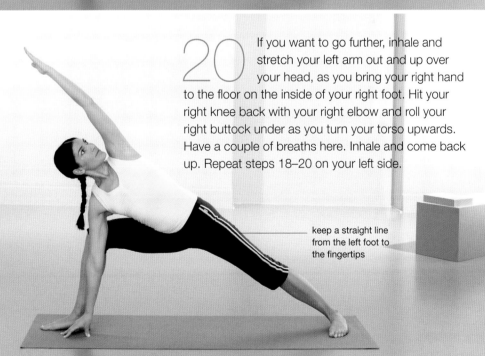

20 If you want to go further, inhale and stretch your left arm out and up over your head, as you bring your right hand to the floor on the inside of your right foot. Hit your right knee back with your right elbow and roll your right buttock under as you turn your torso upwards. Have a couple of breaths here. Inhale and come back up. Repeat steps 18–20 on your left side.

keep a straight line from the left foot to the fingertips

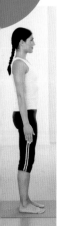

21 Inhale and come back up, bringing your arms down by your side. Stand with your feet hip-width apart, in Mountain Pose (see inset). With your hands on your hips, hinge forward into a Standing Forward Bend. Hold your elbows and release forward. Have a couple of breaths. Inhale and look ahead. Exhale and place your hands on your hips. Inhale and come up with a flat back to Mountain Pose with your arms by your sides.

22 Step your feet together for Tree Pose. Place the sole of your right foot on your inner left thigh. Move your hands into Prayer Position. If you want to go further, inhale and take your arms over your head (see inset). Bring your arms down through the centre line to prayer position. Release your right foot. Bring your feet together and repeat on the other side. If it is difficult to balance, stand next to a wall.

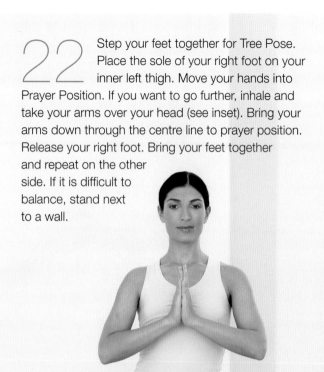

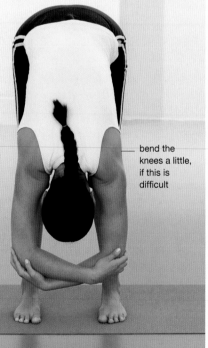

bend the knees a little, if this is difficult

press the foot into the thigh and the thigh into the foot

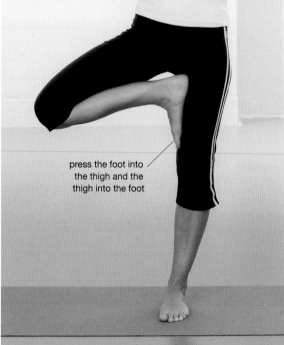

23 Take your chair or stool and place it at the end of the mat. Lie down in front of the chair or stool, with your knees bent towards your chest for a Back Release exercise. Hold your knees with your hands. Exhale and hug your knees towards your chest. Inhale and release. Repeat a couple of times.

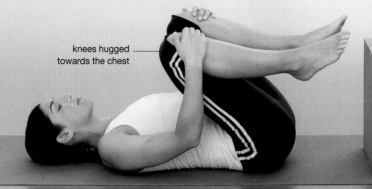

knees hugged towards the chest

24 For the Final Relaxation, bring your arms down by your side and rest your calves on the chair or stool. Check that you are straight and close your eyes. Place a blanket under your head if it is more comfortable, and an eyepad on your eyes. Stay here for 2–5 minutes.

neck is long

palms facing upwards

shoulders relaxed, away from the ears

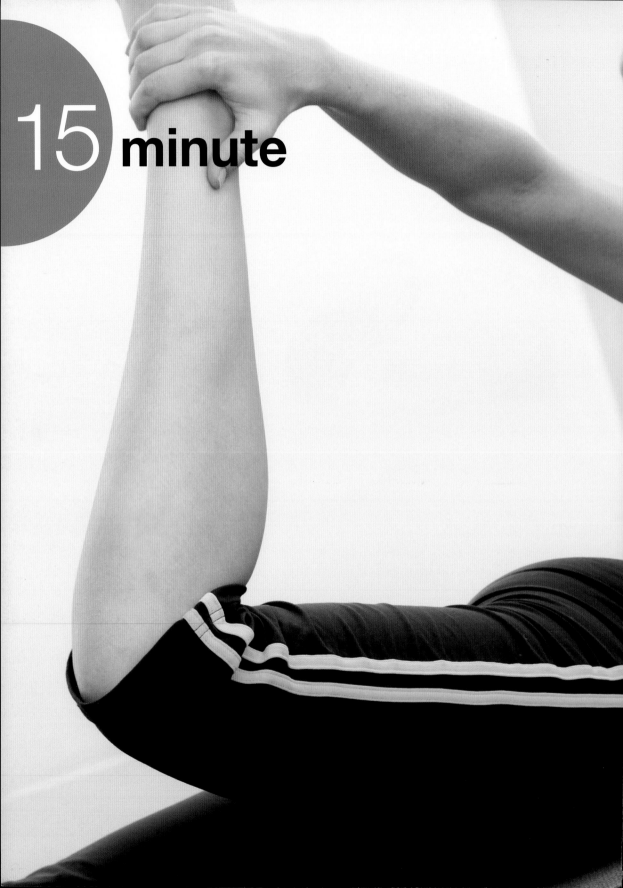

15 minute

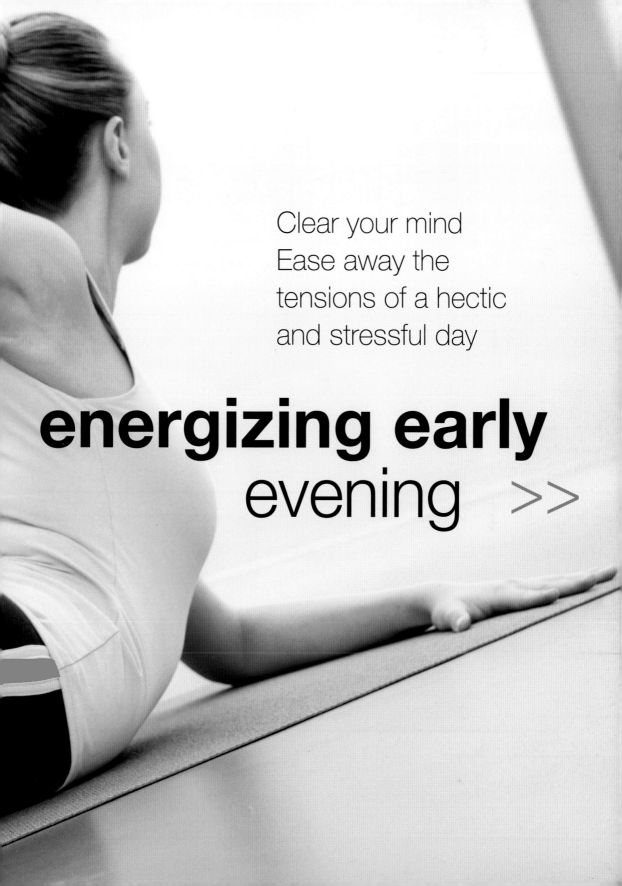

Clear your mind
Ease away the
tensions of a hectic
and stressful day

energizing early
evening >>

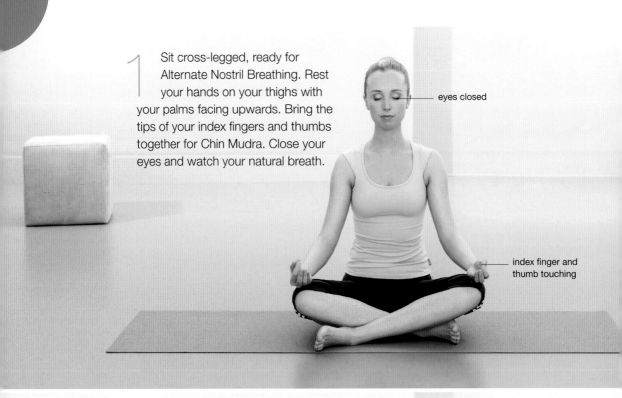

1 Sit cross-legged, ready for Alternate Nostril Breathing. Rest your hands on your thighs with your palms facing upwards. Bring the tips of your index fingers and thumbs together for Chin Mudra. Close your eyes and watch your natural breath.

eyes closed

index finger and thumb touching

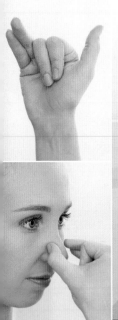

2 On your right hand, bend the index and middle fingers down (see top inset), so that your thumb is free to close your right nostril, and your ring and little fingers are together, ready to close your left nostril. Inhale through both nostrils. Block your right nostril (see bottom inset). Exhale through the left for 4 counts. Inhale through the left for 4 counts. Change, blocking the left nostril. Exhale through the right. Inhale through the right. Change and exhale through the left to complete a full round. Do 2 more rounds.

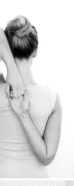

sier option

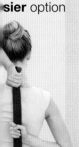

3 Come up to kneeling and bring your arms into Cow Face pose. Take your right hand behind and up your back. Bring your left arm up by your head, bending the elbow so that your forearm comes down your back to clasp the fingers of your right hand. If this is difficult, use a belt (see inset). Feel your abdomen drawing back to the spine to support your lower back. Stay for a couple of breaths. Release your arms and repeat on the other side.

4 Stay kneeling, but tuck your toes under and sit on your heels. Exhale and interlace your fingers, stretching your arms out in front of you. Inhale and lift your arms up over your head, keeping them straight. It is common for the toes to hurt a little here, but you should not experience any knee pain. Stay in this pose for just a few seconds at first.

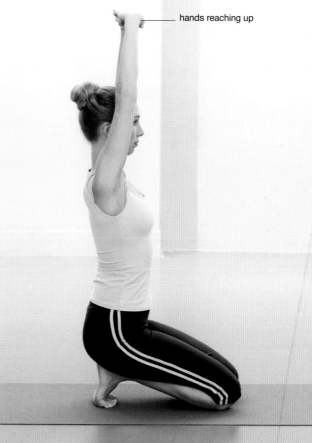

hands reaching up

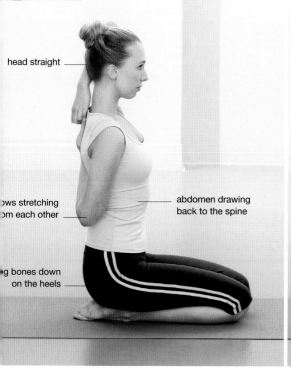

head straight

ws stretching
m each other

abdomen drawing
back to the spine

g bones down
on the heels

>> kneeling pose/shoulder rolls

5 Exhale, releasing your hands. With your left hand on your right thigh and your right hand behind you on your left buttock, twist to the right. Inhale, moving back to the centre. Change the interlace of your fingers and repeat steps 4 and 5, twisting to the left. If your toes are too painful, put your feet flat again and build up gradually to sitting on your heels.

6 Still kneeling, put your feet flat again. Inhale and move your shoulders forward and up. Exhale, moving them back and down. Repeat twice more. Reverse, moving back and up as you inhale and forward and down as you exhale. Repeat twice more.

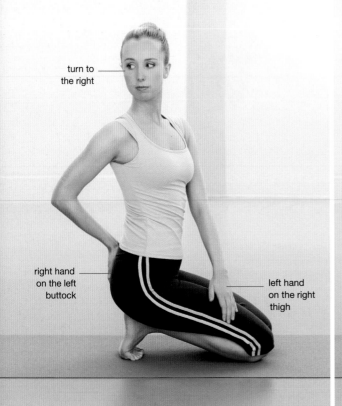

turn to the right

right hand on the left buttock

left hand on the right thigh

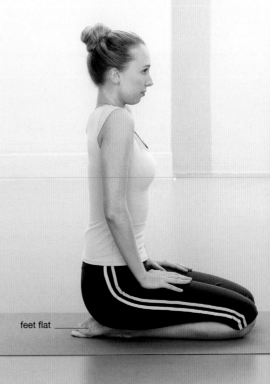

feet flat

7 Come up onto all fours with your hands in line with your shoulders and your knees in line with your hips. Keep your neck long and your shoulders broad and away from your ears. Feel your abdomen drawing back to the spine.

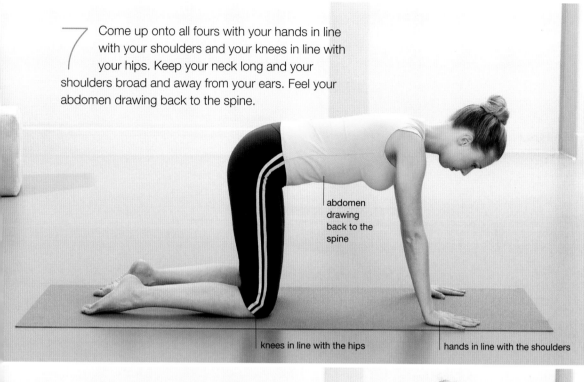

abdomen drawing back to the spine

knees in line with the hips

hands in line with the shoulders

8 Step your right foot forward in between your hands for Lunge. Keep your front shin perpendicular to the floor. If your back knee is hurting on the floor, place a folded towel under it. Sink your hips, stretching your back leg more.

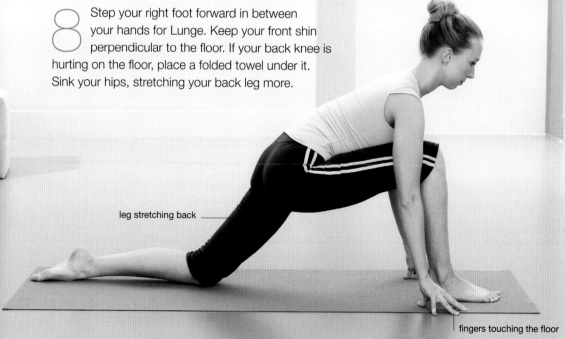

leg stretching back

fingers touching the floor

>> lunge/downward dog

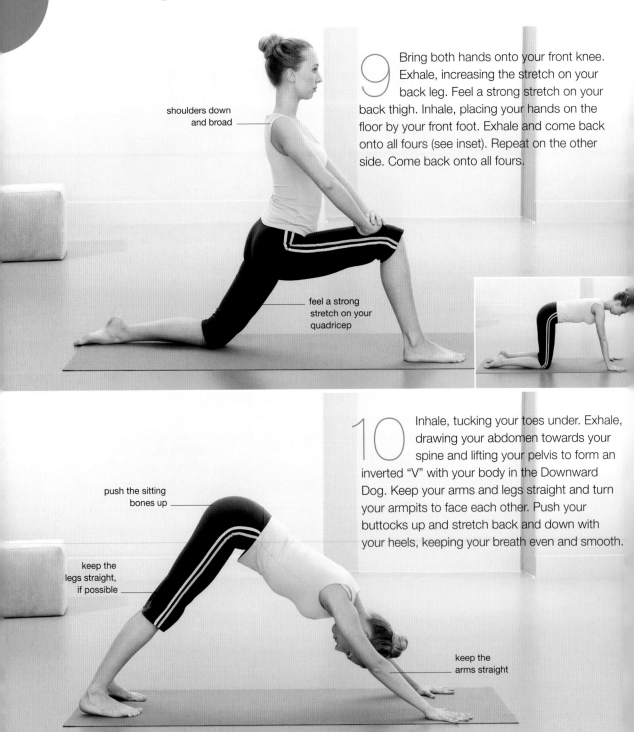

shoulders down
and broad

9 Bring both hands onto your front knee. Exhale, increasing the stretch on your back leg. Feel a strong stretch on your back thigh. Inhale, placing your hands on the floor by your front foot. Exhale and come back onto all fours (see inset). Repeat on the other side. Come back onto all fours.

feel a strong
stretch on your
quadricep

10 Inhale, tucking your toes under. Exhale, drawing your abdomen towards your spine and lifting your pelvis to form an inverted "V" with your body in the Downward Dog. Keep your arms and legs straight and turn your armpits to face each other. Push your buttocks up and stretch back and down with your heels, keeping your breath even and smooth.

push the sitting
bones up

keep the
legs straight,
if possible

keep the
arms straight

>> **diagonal stretch**

11 Inhale and come back onto your knees. Exhale and lie on your stomach with your forehead on the floor and your arms stretched out in front of you.

12 Exhale, lifting and stretching your right arm and left leg and bringing your head just off the floor. Inhale, bring them back down to the floor. Exhale and repeat on your other side. Repeat again on both sides. Make sure you stretch all along the inside of your leg to the heel. As you stretch your arm forward, keep your shoulders away from your ears.

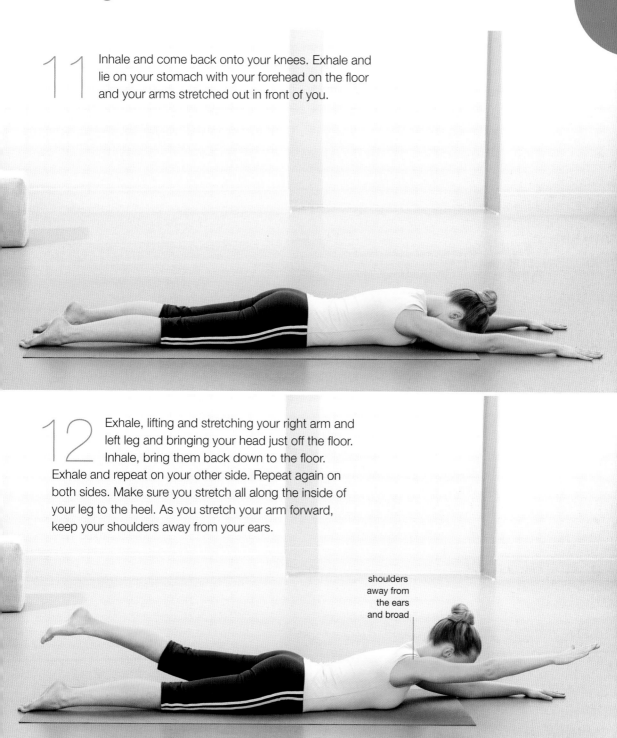

shoulders away from the ears and broad

>> rest/locust

13 Rest. Place your arms by your side with your palms by your hips, facing upwards. Turn your head to one side. Lie with your big toes touching and your heels facing out. Close your eyes and focus on even, gentle breathing.

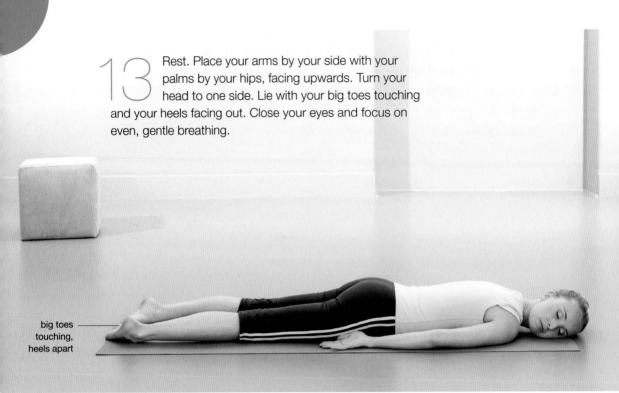

big toes touching, heels apart

14 Inhale, bringing your head back to the centre. Stretch your hands back towards your toes. Keep your feet and legs firmly on the floor as you exhale, peeling your nose, chin, head and shoulders off the floor in the Locust pose. Breathe evenly. As long as there is no pain in your lower back, lift a little higher. Inhale and relax your body down.

keep the neck long

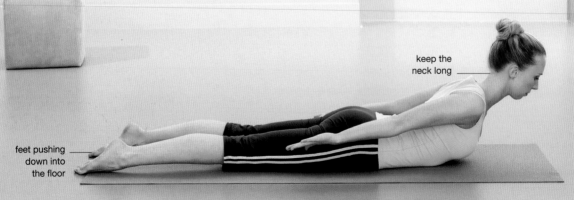

feet pushing down into the floor

15 If you want to work a little harder, exhale, lifting your straight legs as well as your head and shoulders off the floor. Stretch your arms back towards your feet. Inhale and come down. Repeat (as long as you are not experiencing any back pain).

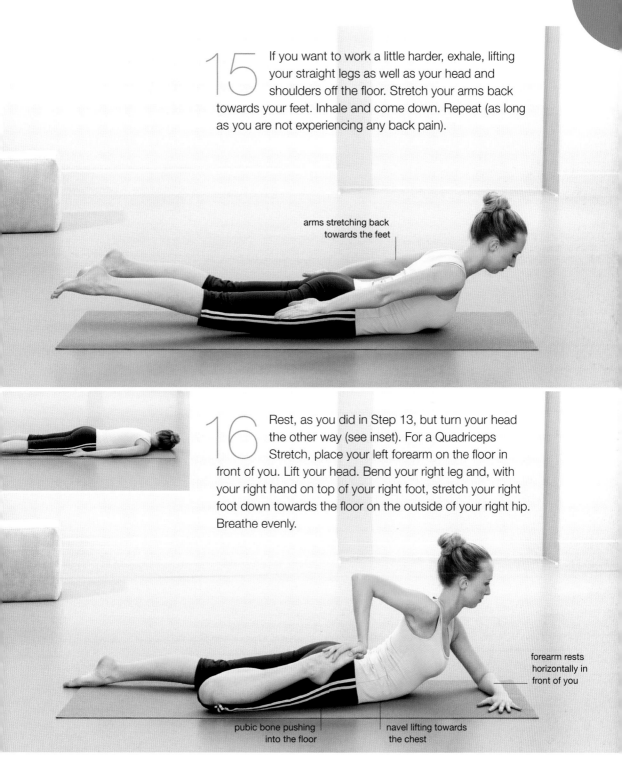

arms stretching back
towards the feet

16 Rest, as you did in Step 13, but turn your head the other way (see inset). For a Quadriceps Stretch, place your left forearm on the floor in front of you. Lift your head. Bend your right leg and, with your right hand on top of your right foot, stretch your right foot down towards the floor on the outside of your right hip. Breathe evenly.

forearm rests
horizontally in
front of you

pubic bone pushing
into the floor

navel lifting towards
the chest

>> half bow/rest

17 Inhale and move your hand to hold the outside of your right ankle, ready for a Half Bow. Keep both hip bones on the floor. Exhale and lift your right thigh up off the floor. Breathe evenly. Inhale and release down. Repeat steps 16 and 17 on your left side.

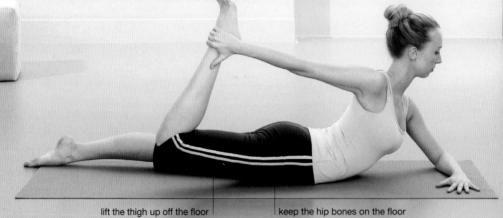

lift the thigh up off the floor | keep the hip bones on the floor

18 Make a pillow with your hands in front of you and rest your forehead on your hands. Lie with your big toes touching and your heels apart. Rest, breathing gently.

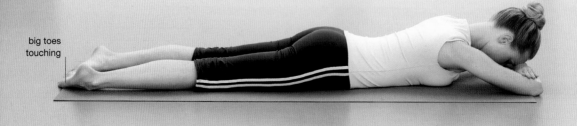

big toes touching

>> full bow/child's pose

easier option

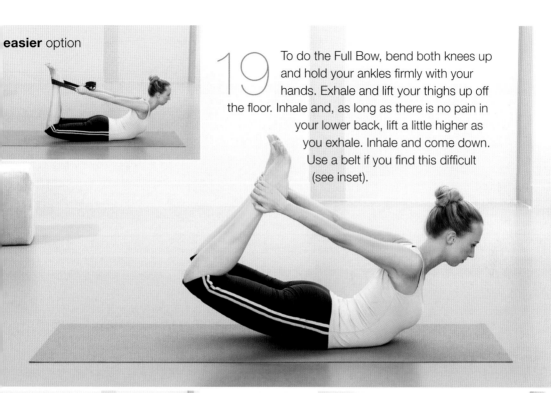

19 To do the Full Bow, bend both knees up and hold your ankles firmly with your hands. Exhale and lift your thighs up off the floor. Inhale and, as long as there is no pain in your lower back, lift a little higher as you exhale. Inhale and come down. Use a belt if you find this difficult (see inset).

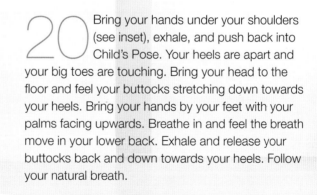

20 Bring your hands under your shoulders (see inset), exhale, and push back into Child's Pose. Your heels are apart and your big toes are touching. Bring your head to the floor and feel your buttocks stretching down towards your heels. Bring your hands by your feet with your palms facing upwards. Breathe in and feel the breath move in your lower back. Exhale and release your buttocks back and down towards your heels. Follow your natural breath.

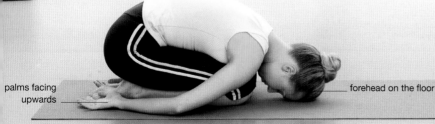

palms facing upwards

forehead on the floor

>> lord of the fishes twist

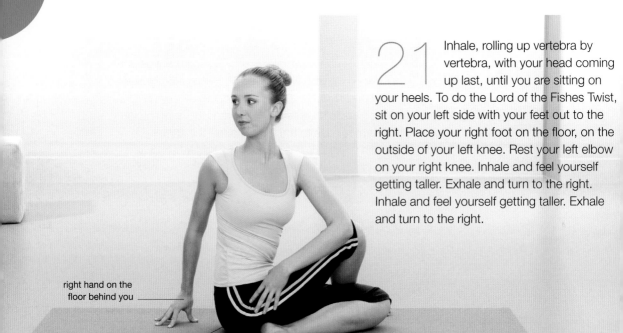

21 Inhale, rolling up vertebra by vertebra, with your head coming up last, until you are sitting on your heels. To do the Lord of the Fishes Twist, sit on your left side with your feet out to the right. Place your right foot on the floor, on the outside of your left knee. Rest your left elbow on your right knee. Inhale and feel yourself getting taller. Exhale and turn to the right. Inhale and feel yourself getting taller. Exhale and turn to the right.

right hand on the floor behind you

sitting bones push down

easier option

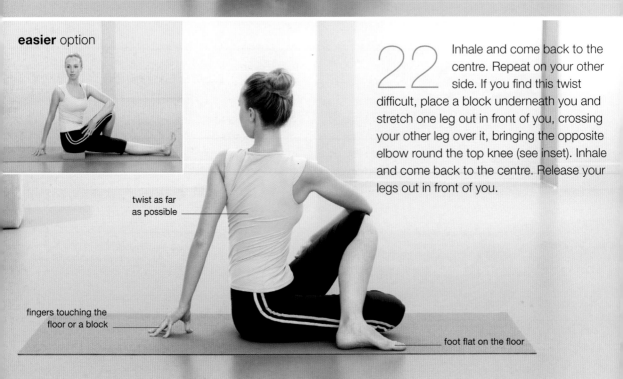

22 Inhale and come back to the centre. Repeat on your other side. If you find this twist difficult, place a block underneath you and stretch one leg out in front of you, crossing your other leg over it, bringing the opposite elbow round the top knee (see inset). Inhale and come back to the centre. Release your legs out in front of you.

twist as far as possible

fingers touching the floor or a block

foot flat on the floor

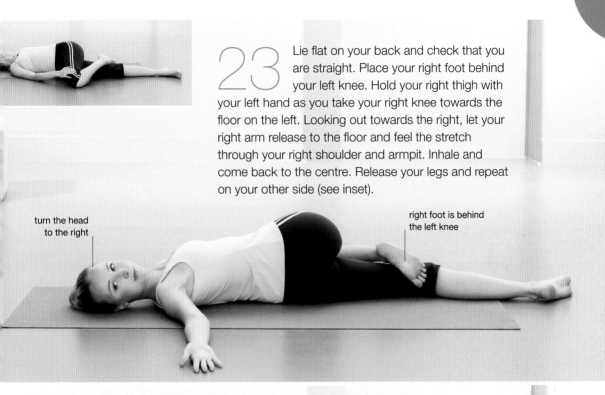

23 Lie flat on your back and check that you are straight. Place your right foot behind your left knee. Hold your right thigh with your left hand as you take your right knee towards the floor on the left. Looking out towards the right, let your right arm release to the floor and feel the stretch through your right shoulder and armpit. Inhale and come back to the centre. Release your legs and repeat on your other side (see inset).

turn the head to the right

right foot is behind the left knee

24 Inhale and come back to the centre. Lie flat with your knees bent and your feet on the floor (hip-width apart and parallel). Lift your head and look down your centre line to see that you are straight. Place your head on the floor and your arms away from your body. Lengthen one leg out along the floor and then the other, ready for the Final Relaxation. Close your eyes and stay here for 2–5 minutes. Place a folded blanket under your head, a cushion under your knees and an eye pad on your eyes, if you wish, to make you more comfortable.

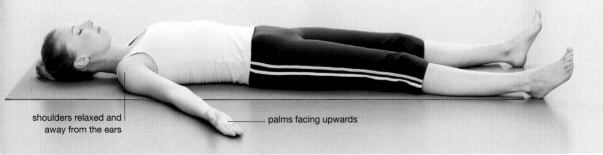

shoulders relaxed and away from the ears

palms facing upwards

index

publisher's acknowledgments

Publisher's acknowledgments

Dorling Kindersley would like to thank project managers Hilary Mandleberg and Helen Murray; project art directors Anne Fisher, Miranda Harvey, and Ruth Hope; photographer Ruth Jenkinson and her assistants Ann Burke, Vic Churchill, and James McNaught; sweatyBetty for the loan of some of the exercise clothing; Viv Riley at Touch Studios; the models Alycea Ungaro and Charlie Arnaldo in *Everyday Pilates*, Jacqui Freeman and Carla Collins in *Abs Workout*, Rhona Crewe and Sam Johannesson in *Better Back Workout,* Kerry Jay and Samantha Johannesson in *Total Body Workout*, and Tara Lee and Susan Reynolds in *Gentle Yoga*; Victoria Barnes and Roisin Donaghy for the models' hair and makeup; YogaMatters for the loan of the mat and other equipment; Hilary Bird for the index; Claire Tennant-Scull for proofreading; Robert Sharman, Susannah Marriott, Andrea Bagg, and Tara Woolnough for editorial assistance; and Elma Aquino and Danaya Bunnag for design assistance.

DVD credits

Dorling Kindersley would like to thank directors Joel Mishcon, Gez Medinger, Robin Schmidt, and Sami Abusamra; producer Hannah Chandler; DOPs Marcus Domleo, Benedict Spence, and Matthew Cooke; Benedict Spence, Joe McNally, Marcus Domleo, and Jonathan Iles on the camera; gaffers Paul Wilcox, Johann Cruickshank, and Jonathan Spencer; grips Pete Nash and Terry Williams; production manager Hannah Chandler; production assistants Nathan Nikolov, Irene Maffei, Azra Gul, Tom Robinson, and Krisztina Fenyvesi; Chad Hobson and Scott Shields for music; Roisin Donaghy and Victoria Barnes for hair and makeup; Suzanne Pirret and Alycea Ungaro for voiceover work; and Ben Jones and Charles de Montebello (CDM Studios) for voiceover recording.

Picture credits

All images © Dorling Kindersley
For further information see: www.dkimages.com

about the authors

Joan Pagano

Joan Pagano is certified in health and fitness instruction by the American College of Sports Medicine (ACSM). She has worked as a personal fitness trainer on Manhattan's Upper East Side since 1988. Today, Joan manages her own staff of trainers in the Joan Pagano Fitness Group and is a nationally recognized provider of education courses for fitness trainers as well as an authority on the benefit of exercise for women's health issues. She is the author of several books. To learn more, visit www.joanpaganofitness.com.

Alycea Ungaro

Alycea Ungaro, PT, is the owner of Alycea Ungaro's Real Pilates in New York City and the author of several best-selling Pilates titles. Alycea's personal mission is to make Pilates available to everyone regardless of age, fitness level, or geographic location. To that end, Alycea has created Pilates products in every possible medium. She presents seminars and workshops nationally and also serves on the advisory board of Fitness Magazine. Alycea is a featured personality on Nextfit.com and iamplify.com, where you can download her signature workouts to your desktop or iPod. She lives in New York City with her family. To learn more about Alycea, visit www.alyceaungaro.com. To find out about Real Pilates, visit www.realpilatesnyc.com.

Louise Grime

Louise teaches hatha yoga in London, mainly at Triyoga in Primrose Hill and Soho and at The Life Centre, Notting Hill Gate. She started practicing yoga with Silvia Prescott and Penny Neild-Smith, two of the first Iyengar teachers in London, in 1978. Since then, she has spent time in the Sivananda Ashram in Kerala, India, where she completed teachers' training and advanced teachers' training. In 1994, Louise qualified as an Iyengar yoga teacher in London. Louise takes a keen interest in Eastern and Western spiritual traditions and meditation. When teaching she likes to incorporate the yogic philosophy into her classes.

Suzanne Martin

Suzanne is a doctor of physical therapy and a Pilates expert. A former dancer, she is certified as a Master trainer by the American Council on Exercise and is well known in both the US and Europe as an educational presenter in Pilates, dance, and physical therapy. Suzanne is the lead physical therapist for the Smuin Ballet in San Francisco and maintains a private practice, Total Body Development, in Alameda, California. She is also educational director for Pilates Therapeutics LLC, devoted to the therapeutic application of the Pilates Method, and her Pilates Therapeutics® educational videos are available on DVD and as downloads on iamplify.com. For more information, go to www.totalbodydevelopment.com and pilatestherapeutics.com.